推拿
Tui na

by the same author

Chinese Massage Manual
A comprehensive, step-by-step introduction
to the healing art of Tui na
Sarah Pritchard
Foreword by Li He
ISBN 978 0 95629 300 8
eISBN 978 0 85701 217 3

of related interest

Tuina/Massage Manipulations
Basic Principles and Technique
Chief Editor: Li Jiangshan
ISBN 978 1 84819 058 0
eISBN 978 0 85701 046 9

Elemental Bodywork (Tuina)
Assessment and Application of Chinese
Massage through the Five Elements
Thomas Droge
ISBN 978 1 84819 244 7
eISBN 978 0 85701 189 3

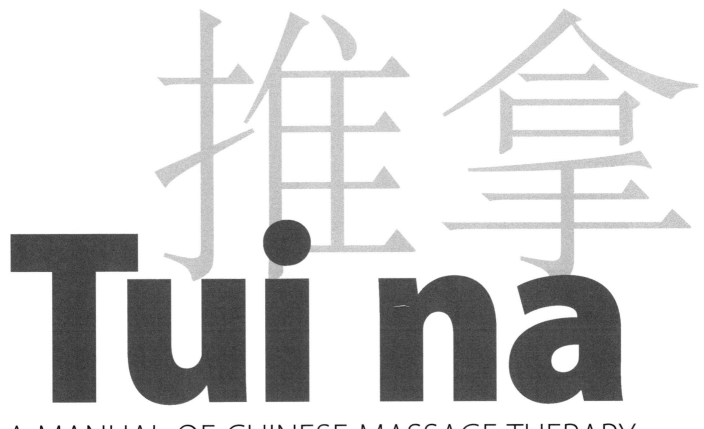

Tui na

A MANUAL OF CHINESE MASSAGE THERAPY

Sarah Pritchard

Dip Tui na Clin.cert Tui na (Nanjing) Lic. Ac. MBAcC

Tui na Course Coordinator and Senior Lecturer,
City College of Acupuncture, London;
Director, Blackheath Complementary Health Centre, London, UK;
Practitioner of Acupuncture, Tui na and Reiki

With a Contribution by Andrew Croysdale Dip Tui na MGCP MRCMT
Lecturer and Tui na Clinical Supervisor,
London College of Traditional Acupuncture and Oriental Medicine, London

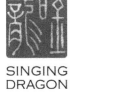

SINGING
DRAGON
LONDON AND PHILADELPHIA

This edition published in 2015
by Singing Dragon
an imprint of Jessica Kingsley Publishers
73 Collier Street
London N1 9BE, UK
and
400 Market Street, Suite 400
Philadelphia, PA 19106, USA

www.singingdragon.com

First published in 2010 by Elsevier Ltd

Library of Congress Cataloging in Publication Data
A CIP catalog record for this book is available from the Library of Congress

British Library Cataloguing in Publication Data
A CIP catalogue record for this book is available from the British Library

ISBN 978 1 84819 269 0
eISBN 978 0 85701 218 0

Printed and bound in Great Britain

Contents

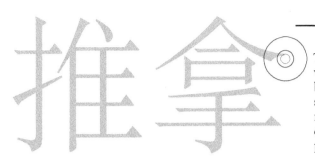

There are videos which accompany this text including video sequences of all the techniques indicated in the text by the icon. These videos are available at www. singingdragon.com/catalogue/book/9781848192690/ resources. The videos are designed to be used in conjunction with the text and not as a stand-alone product.

Section Three Tui na treatment – general principles for creating and planning treatments

Tui na, or Chinese massage therapy, is one of the four main branches of traditional Chinese medicine. However, though its roots in China are ancient, it is still relatively new to the West. Archaeological studies have dated the use of Chinese massage therapy back to around 3000BC, making it the grandmother of all forms of massage and body work that exist today, from shiatsu to osteopathy, and the first form of Chinese medicine practiced.

Given this history, its popularity in China and the breadth of its therapeutic ability, it is perhaps surprising that it was the last branch of Chinese medicine to be recognized in the West.

I am glad that this situation is changing rapidly. When I was studying in the early 1990s, very few people in the UK and indeed throughout the West knew what Tui na was, and there was very little training available. Over the past 10 years this has been changing. Now, more colleges of Chinese medicine in the West have begun to offer Tui na practitioner training courses alongside their acupuncture and herbal medicine programs. It seems that Tui na is now entering another period of flourishing and development; this time in the West.

A recent survey conducted by the British Acupuncture Council about its members revealed that Tui na is now the most popular form of treatment for practitioners to use in conjunction with acupuncture. This shows a remarkable growth in the interest and popularity of Tui na among acupuncturists in the UK.

Many people in the West have been drawn to and helped by Chinese herbal medicine and acupuncture. As the popularity of Tui na spreads, more people will reap the benefits of this therapy, as they have done in China for thousands of years.

Tui na differs from other forms of massage in that it is used to treat specific illnesses of an internal nature as well as muscular skeletal ailments. Becoming a Tui na practitioner is a rewarding, if demanding process. You need a thorough knowledge of the theoretical principles of Chinese medicine and its channel system and points, a knowledge of Western anatomy, physiology and pathology, and the ability to perform a range of manual techniques according to your diagnosis.

This book is a comprehensive foundation textbook for students and practitioners of Tui na to help them with the process of acquiring the necessary manual skills and for developing the art of applying Tui na to adult patients. I hope this book will also be useful to acupuncturists and to practitioners of other forms of Oriental medicine and bodywork who are interested in learning Tui na. I have not covered infantile Tui na in this book – this specialized branch of Tui na deals with the treatment of children under 7 years and I hope to cover this in a future book.

This book contains a detailed section on Tui na techniques including their clinical application and therapeutic effects. I believe in an integrated approach to Tui na and I have included information and examples of yin and yang styles of practice. There are also chapters on external herbal massage media and ancillary therapies. The final section of the book focuses on creating and planning Tui na treatments and how to apply them. Instead of using prescribed treatments I encourage you to formulate your own and I have given suggestions and guidelines, illustrated by many cases from my own practice.

Through my own experience of studying, practicing and teaching Tui na, I have discovered that there is always more to learn. As a student I learnt from my teachers, as a practitioner I learn from my patients, and as a teacher I learn from my students.

I hope this book helps you on the way to becoming an effective Tui na practitioner and encourages further progression and development of Tui na in the West.

Sarah Pritchard
London 2010

SECTION ONE

Foundations

CHAPTER **1**

Foundations and development of Tui na

A brief history of Tui na

Tui na has a long history with many periods of flourishing and development. The first massage techniques were born instinctively from the needs of the people who were living physically hard lives, exposed to the elements and prone to frequent injuries. They discovered that An (*pressing*) would stop bleeding and Mo (*rubbing*) would ease pain and reduce swelling. Evidence from archaeological digs suggests that massage was first practiced over 3000 years ago. Ancient oracle bones and tortoise shells were discovered upon which there are inscriptions that refer to a female shaman known as a Bi who cured people with massage. Medicine was inseparable from ritual life and was directed and developed by the shamans of the time who became the first doctors. Massage became quite sophisticated even in these early times.

In the late Zhou dynasty (700–481 BC), texts on the development of Chinese medicine refer to massage or 'An Wu', as it was then called. These texts mention various techniques including the compound techniques. There is also mention of a famous Dr Bian Que working with a combination of massage and acupuncture. At the same time there are records of widespread folk use of massage therapy in the writing of the philosophers of the time such as Lao Zi (reputed author of the 'Dao De Jing').

A ten-volume work specifically on massage called 'Huangdi Qibo Anmo Shijuan' *Classics on Massage of the Yellow Emperor and Qi Bo* attributed to the Qin dynasty (221–207 BC) was the first detailed work of its kind. Unfortunately this classic of massage was lost. It came out at the same time as 'Huangdi Neijing' *Classic of Internal Medicine of the Yellow Emperor*, which mainly recorded the theory of Chinese medicine and the use of acupuncture but did also include several chapters and sections devoted to massage therapy, including descriptions of 12 techniques and their therapeutic effects and clinical applications.

The next important reference to Chinese massage therapy is by one of China's great medical geniuses, Zhang Zhong Jing (AD 142–220) who lived during the later Han dynasty (AD 25–220). He was possibly the world's first medical specialist, having a special interest in febrile diseases. His contribution was to establish the principles of drug combining, one of the great achievements of Chinese herbal medicine. He applied these principles to the use of herbal ointments in massage therapy to increase the therapeutic effects. This process was called Gao mo (*ointment massage*). Hua Tuo, another famous doctor of the time and China's first recorded surgeon, mentions Gao mo applied for expelling pathogenic factors that had invaded the Exterior. Gao mo continued to develop and grow in popularity and several texts were written on its uses, including prescriptions for making ointments and the diseases that they could treat.

During the Sui (AD 589–618) and Tang (AD 618–906) dynasties, massage therapy really started to flourish. A department of massage therapy was founded within the Office of Imperial Physicians and the practice and teaching of Chinese massage therapy blossomed. There was an experienced massage doctor in charge of the daily treatments and teaching who worked with a team of massage practitioners and massage workers. Massage treatment and the teaching of students were promoted. The work done during this time laid the foundations for what would become modern Tui na.

Dr Sun Si Miao (AD 590–682) who worked during this period introduced a further 10 massage techniques in his book *The Massage of Lao Zi* and for the first time systemized the treatment of childhood diseases using massage therapy. One special technique that he pioneered was the application of external herbal media on points to treat and prevent disease in children. In his book *Six Classics in the Tang Dynasty* he describes the treatment of diseases caused by Wind, Cold, Damp and Heat, Deficiency and Excess, with massage therapy. It was during this period that massage therapy took its place as a medical treatment in its own right alongside acupuncture and herbal medicine.

Also during this period Chinese massage therapy began to spread to other countries, initially to Japan, where by AD702 the study of massage became compulsory for all medical students. Then with China's strong cultural influences it spread to other countries including Korea and Vietnam and via the silk trade route to the lands of Islam.

In the Song dynasty (AD960–1279) and the Yuan dynasty (AD1280–1368), an intensive analysis of Chinese massage techniques was undertaken and the therapy was further refined. It became the primary form of treatment in the bone-setting and pediatric departments at the Institute of Imperial Physicians. During this time there was much importance placed on analyzing the massage techniques.

The Ming dynasty (AD1368–1644) saw the second great flourishing of massage therapy. It was during this time that it took the name Tui na after two of the most common manipulations and partly because the term 'Anmo' had become associated with prostitution. Many texts were written during this period, particularly on pediatric Tui na, which had become hugely popular. Tui na specialists from all over China met to discuss diagnosis, techniques and treatments.

During the Qing dynasty (AD1644–1912), Tui na continued to develop and thrive in both imperial and public domains.

In the early part of the 20th century, traditional Chinese medicine (TCM) began to suffer greatly. This was due to competition from the mainly symptomatic treatments of Western medicine now available. There was, in fact, a time when it looked like TCM would die out completely. Between 1912 and 1948, during the rule of Guo Min Dang, doctors trained in Western medicine returned to China from Japan and recommended that TCM be banned. Fortunately, this was rejected at the National Medical Assembly in Shanghai on 17 March 1929, thanks to massive lobbying. This day is remembered each year and celebrated as Chinese Doctors' Day.

However, the battle was not over. Mao Ze Dong was also against TCM until the Long March of 1934–1935. There were no drugs, anesthetics or surgery available, and doctors of TCM came to the rescue, achieving amazing results with vast numbers of wounded and sick soldiers.

From this time on, TCM had its feet planted firmly on the ground of modern medicine and, under the People's Republic of China established in 1948, all departments of TCM were nurtured and encouraged to grow. In 1956, the first official training course in Tui na was opened in Shanghai; other hospitals followed suit and by 1974 Tui na training departments had been set up all over China. By 1978, whole hospitals were devoted to the practice of TCM and all other hospitals held within them special TCM

departments. International training centers for TCM were established in Beijing, Nanjing, Shanghai, Anhui, Zhejiang and Shandong. In 1987, the Chinese National Tui Na Association was established which holds regular meetings for Tui na doctors to share their clinical experiences and offer papers on their work.

The UK Register of Tui na Chinese Massage has recently been set up in order to promote high standards of training and practice, to encourage practitioners to share their experiences of applying Tui na in the treatment of Western patients and to promote the development and public awareness of Tui na in the UK.

The famous schools of Tui na

Many different schools of Tui na developed in China, each with its own particular style, strength and therapeutic effects. As with Qigong, numerous forms of Tui na developed within particular families and communities, especially in the remote areas of China. These family styles developed from the health needs of the local people and were passed down originally by the local shamans and then through families for generations.

Out of the many and varied approaches, five Tui na schools became particularly famous. These five schools, all of which have had a significant influence on the application of modern Tui na, are:

1. Yi zhi chan tui fa: one-finger meditation school
2. Gun fa: rolling school
3. An fa: point pressure school
4. Ji dian fa: striking school
5. Neigong: internal exercise school

Yi zhi chan tui fa: one-finger meditation school

This school originated and developed in the Qing dynasty (1644–1911). It uses Yi zhi chan tui fa as the primary technique and makes use of a further 11 supporting techniques which are: Na fa (*grasping*), An fa (*pressing*), Gun fa (*rolling*), Mo fa (*round rubbing*), Nian fa (*holding–twisting*), Cuo fa (*rub rolling*), Tui fa (*pushing*), Rou fa (*kneading*), Yao fa (*rotating*), Duo fa (*shaking*) and Ma fa (*wiping*).

The techniques are applied powerfully but softly and are penetrating in their effect. The chief manipulation is difficult to learn and master so great attention and importance are given to basic training exercises, Shaolin sinew changing Qigong and continuous practice of the difficult techniques on rice bags.

This school emphasizes the stimulation of groups of prescribed points and sections of channels. It is used to treat an extensive range of diseases and specializes in the treatment of ailments that are related to internal disharmonies such as headaches, dizziness, insomnia, hypertension, menstrual disorders, digestive problems and lower backache.

Gun fa: rolling school

The rolling school developed in the 1940s out of the one-finger meditation school. The primary technique applied is Gun fa (*rolling*) and the supportive techniques are Na fa (*grasping*) and the compound versions of Na fa, An fa (*pressing*), Nian fa (*holding–twisting*), Cuo fa (*rub rolling*) and Rou fa (*kneading*). Techniques are often coordinated and applied simultaneously with passive movements of the joints. Techniques are applied to points, along channels and to joints. The training required is the same as for the one-finger meditation school. Rolling produces a soft rhythmic stimulation of the body; it has a large manipulating area and a powerful ability to move Qi. This school specializes in the treatment of diseases of the nervous system, all forms of paralysis, headache, joint injuries, chronic joint disease and soft tissue injuries such as muscle sprains.

An fa: point pressure school

This is the oldest school, originally developed by the ancient shamans and strongly linked with the practice of folk medicine throughout the historical development of Chinese massage therapy. A reference from the 'Huang Di Neijing' states that 'pressing can resolve Blood stasis, dispel qi and relieve pain, pressing produces heat and heat can relieve pain'.

The primary technique employed is An fa (*pressing*), which is often combined with Rou fa (*kneading*) or applied as the compound technique pushing–pressing. Zhen fa (*vibrating*) and Na fa (*grasping*) are used as supportive techniques.

This school emphasizes the stimulation of points and channels with pressure that is applied with the thumbs, fingers, elbows, palms and forearms. It has a wide therapeutic range and is effective for regulating the flow of Qi and Blood, dredging the channels, harmonizing and tonifying the Zangfu, dispersing Cold and stagnation of Qi and Blood and relieving pain.

Ji dian fa: striking school

This school, which is particularly popular in the Shandong province, is linked with traditional Chinese martial arts and evolved from the An fa point pressure school.

The primary technique is Ji dian fa (*digital striking*). The supportive techniques employed are Pai fa (*knocking*), Ji fa (*chopping*), An fa (*pressing*) and compound versions of Na fa (*grasping*). The application of the techniques is swift and energetic.

Practitioners have to develop strong fingers and arms and good supporting power from the legs to practice this form. It is commonly used by martial arts practitioners to deal with injuries and to correct the flow of Qi. This form is effective for dredging channels, promoting the flow of Qi and Blood, regulating Wei and Ying Qi, tonifying Qi and expelling pathogens.

Neigong: internal exercise school

The emphasis of training is on the cultivation of internal Qi. Practitioners train in Shaolin internal Qigong and develop the ability to direct Qi along the channels and inside the patient's body. The primary technique is Tui fa (*pushing*) and this is supported by a variety of other techniques, especially Zhen fa (*vibrating*); compound versions of Rou fa (*kneading*) and Na fa (*grasping*). Techniques are performed in the typical Northern Chinese style: vigorously, powerfully and briskly; but within their application is softness and smoothness. Gentleness (Yin) and strength (Yang) are equally balanced.

The approach of the internal Qi school is always to treat the whole body. Techniques are applied in routine sequences that cover the head, face, back, chest, abdomen and the four limbs. The routine is altered subtly according to the individual patient's patterns of disharmony.

This school specializes in the treatment of internal disharmony, nourishing the Zangfu, clearing pathogens and strengthening the Wei Qi.

The influence of all of these schools can be seen in the practice of Tui na today. Training in the TCM colleges in China is based for the most part on a combination of the one-finger meditation, rolling and Neigong schools.

Chinese massage therapy has always evolved with the times, the environment and the health needs of the people. In the West, the training and practice of Tui na is continuing to develop and evolve to suit the health needs of Western patients. Practitioners in the West need a flexible approach to deal with the demands of the times. This has led to the beginnings of a further integration of aspects of the five famous Chinese schools, some approaches from the family systems and the blending of Yin and Yang styles.

How Tui na works

Tui na has the ability to:

- Promote and invigorate the flow of Qi and Blood
- Expel, clear, dissipate and dredge pathogenic factors
- Regulate Qi and Blood
- Harmonize Yin and Yang, Wei Qi and Ying Qi
- Nourish, tonify, strengthen and support Qi and Blood, Yin and Yang
- Improve and regulate the functions of the Zangfu
- Release and relax the channel sinews
- Lubricate and facilitate the movement of joints
- Soothe Qi and calm the Shen

Tui na achieves the above by stimulating the points, channels and collaterals appropriate to the presenting disharmony with manual massage techniques, passive movements, directed Qi and intention. Tui na works by combining the following:

- The rationale and principles of Chinese medicine
- The therapeutic qualities of the Tui na techniques
- The method of applying the techniques
- The practitioner's intention and ability to direct their awareness and Qi through their hands

A physical therapy and a form of Qigong energy medicine

Tui na is both a form of physical bodywork and a subtle energy medicine. As a physical therapy it excels at releasing the channel sinews, (collectively the muscles, tendons and ligaments) and facilitating the movement of joints.

By opening, releasing and balancing the channel sinews, Tui na is able to treat not only muscular skeletal problems, but also any ailment that may be caused by emotional and postural holding patterns that have become unconscious and locked into the body's protective connective tissue armour.

As a form of energy medicine or Qigong, practitioners utilize and direct Qi through their hands, into points, along channels and into the Zangfu and bones. Tui na can be very vigorous and physically active or incredibly subtle and still. It depends on the style of the practitioner and the requirements of treatment.

Application of the rationale and principles of Chinese medicine

As with acupuncture and Chinese herbal medicine, Tui na is inseparable from the rationale and philosophy of Chinese medicine. In order to choose the most appropriate Tui na techniques to apply and where and how to apply them, the practitioner must be able to make a diagnosis according to its principles. Without this, Tui na has no context and cannot be therapeutically effective. It would be like teaching an acupuncturist to insert and manipulate a needle and no more.

The combination of the practitioner's clear intention, their ability to choose and apply suitable Tui na techniques and direct their attention and Qi, makes Tui na a versatile and effective form of treatment for a wide range of diseases.

Therapeutic qualities of the Tui na techniques

Each technique has its own therapeutic qualities. When performed correctly for an appropriate length of time, each technique creates its own particular wave signal or vibratory pattern. These rhythmic waves and vibrations can affect the Qi on all levels, traveling through points and along the channels and collaterals to the desired place.

Method of application

Techniques can be applied in a variety of ways depending on the principle of treatment. For example, the technique Rou fa (*kneading*), applied with the palm of the hand gently, slowly and in a clockwise direction for 5 minutes over the point Zhongwan Ren12 will tonify and warm the Stomach and Spleen. The same technique applied vigorously, briskly and in an anti-clockwise direction at a sinew channel binding area will release and relax the muscles, tendons and ligaments, and move stagnant Qi and Blood.

The practitioner's intention and ability to work with Qi

A clear intention and the ability to gently direct conscious attention is a powerful therapeutic tool. Some forms of Yin-style Tui na such as bone-holding and pulsing are essentially based on this ability and the law of human resonance. In Chinese medicine the treatment principle provides the practitioner with a clear intention. With the intention formed in the practitioner's mind, they can then allow a connection to be made with the unlimited field of healing information available in the universe. This universal Qi can then be utilized and directed through the practitioner's hands and into points, channels, organs, bones and so on.

Becoming an effective Tui na practitioner – training requirements and practitioner cultivation

Learning and practicing Tui na is a challenging and rewarding process. To become a good Tui na practitioner you must have a comprehensive knowledge and understanding of Chinese medicine theory, the channel system and the location, nature and actions of the points. You need to be able to apply this knowledge to make a diagnosis and combine this with your knowledge of the therapeutic qualities of the Tui na techniques in order to create a treatment.

You also need to develop your strength, flexibility, stamina and coordination and to cultivate your Qi so that you can become both manually proficient at applying the Tui na techniques and therapeutically effective by learning to direct Qi through your hands.

Qigong

Some form of Qigong practice is essential for Tui na students and practitioners. All good courses will include Qigong as part of the training program. There are many different forms and styles of Qigong, all with their own benefits. Colleges offering Tui na training will vary in the form of Qigong that they teach; it often depends on the emphasis of the style of Tui na being taught. Many of you may already be practicing Qigong and will already be familiar with the benefits of regular practice.

Traditionally, the first system of Qigong most commonly taught to Tui na students is Shaolin Neigong. It is particularly well suited to the development of Tui na practitioners because it is one of the most effective methods for strengthening the channel sinews, developing stamina and cultivating Wei Qi. It is taught to students during the first part of their training when they are learning how to practice and apply the Tui na techniques. This is the system of Qigong that I was initially taught during my training and I encourage students to learn this system. If you practice regularly it will strengthen your resistance to disease, you will feel stronger, more energetic and vital and it will help you to master the Tui na techniques that are more difficult to acquire such as Zhen fa, Yi zhi chan tui fa and Gun fa. Traditionally, other forms of Qigong such as six sounds Qigong are introduced later on in Tui na training. It is beyond the scope of this book to go into detail about the practice of Qigong and I refer you to the bibliography and resources section at the back of this book for further reading and information about courses and classes.

I have included below a few simple but powerful exercises that I have found to be particularly useful to use on a day-to-day basis for relaxing, grounding and centering, for expanding and protecting the energy field, for drawing down universal Qi, focusing the mind, developing Qi awareness in the hands and for cleansing and clearing after a day of treatments.

Grounding and centering energy (Fig. 1.1)

When you work with patients you need to feel connected to the Earth and centered, balanced and relaxed within yourself.

All touch-based therapies make use of the law of resonance; so if you are in a calm, grounded and comfortable state this will resonate through to your patient. I recommend that you get into the habit of grounding, centering and protecting your energy by practicing these exercises before you practice your Tui na techniques. If you do, your practice time will be more focused and efficient and by the time you come to work with patients these practices will be second nature.

Grounding

Stand with your feet shoulder width apart, knees slightly bent. Close your eyes and relax your body. Scan your body

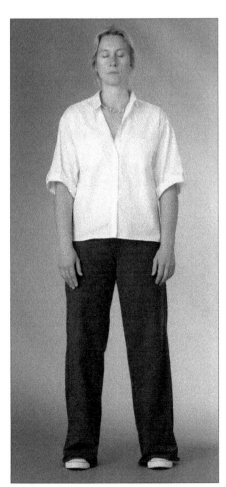

Fig. 1.1 Grounding and centering.

for any areas of tension and holding, bring your attention and breath to these areas and ask them to release. Bring your attention to Yongquan KD1 and imagine these points at the soles of your feet opening like trap doors. Visualize tree roots moving out of the trap doors and down into the Earth, becoming stronger and thicker as they descend to a place in the center of the Earth where they connect and bind. These are your grounding roots, connecting you to the Yin energy of the Earth. As you inhale, imagine drawing your breath in from the center of the Earth, up through your roots, up the Yin channels of your legs and into your Dantian. As you exhale allow the breath to descend back down through your roots and into the Earth. Do this until you feel a strong magnetic sense of connection with the Earth. Say the word 'grounded' to yourself three times.

Centering

Put the tip of your tongue at the roof of your mouth just behind your teeth. Imagine a pearl in your lower abdomen in the center of your Dantian, bring your mental attention to the pearl and breathe into it. Deliberately extend your breaths so that they become deeper and longer and imagine the pearl glowing brighter with each breath. Say the word 'centered' to yourself three times.

Protection

Five-element protection and the pillar of light (Fig. 1.2)

This is a very powerful Qigong meditation that was used in ancient times by doctors and practitioners before they went to treat patients in epidemic situations. It will help to protect you from external pathogenic factors and from absorbing any pathogenic Qi that may be released from patients during treatment. If you work in a big city as I do, it is easy to feel pushed along by the urgent electric city energy. I find this exercise recharges my batteries, helps me to maintain my own rhythm and to feel a sense of space around me. Proceed as follows:

- Stand or sit facing south and close your eyes. Bring your attention to the pearl in your Dantian and breathe into it nine times.
- Bring your attention to your liver, breathe into your liver and imagine green mist filling it, allow this mist to expand from your liver through to the left side of your body then beyond your body to fill the eastern quarter as far as you can imagine into the horizon to your left. Visualize the green mist turning into a vast, deep green forest dense with trees. See the forest expanding as far and as wide as you can imagine into the eastern horizon. Visualize a great green dragon, the guardian of the wood element, flying over the forest.
- Breathe once into the pearl in your Dantian.
- Bring your attention to your lungs, breathe into your lungs and imagine a white mist filling them. Allow this mist to expand through to the right side of your body and fill the western quarter as far as you can imagine into the horizon on your right-hand side.

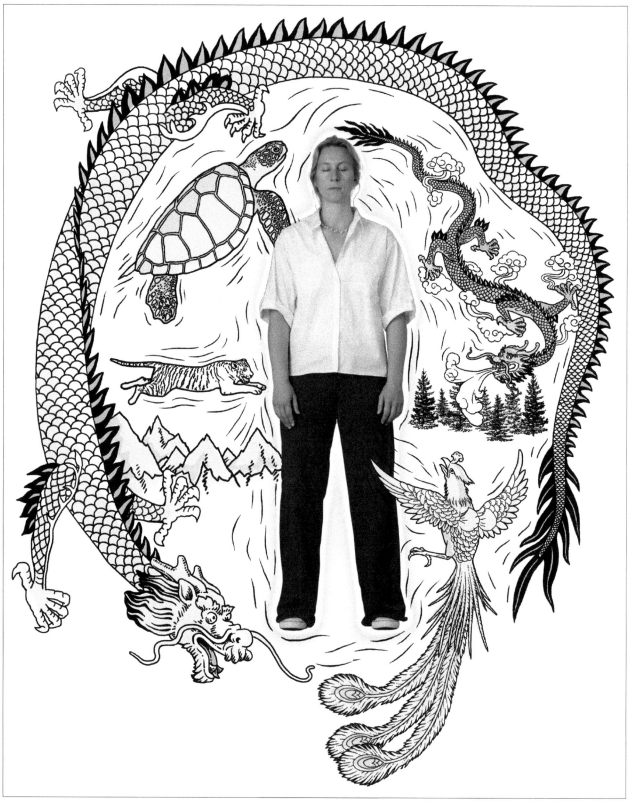

Fig. 1.2 Protection: five-element protection exercise.

Visualize the white mist turning into a massive range of iron ore mountains covered with snow and with snow all around. See the mountains expanding far and wide into the western horizon. Visualize a huge white tiger, the guardian of the Metal Element, leaping from mountain to mountain.

- Breathe once into the pearl in your Dantian.
- Bring your attention to your heart, breathe into your heart and imagine a red mist filling your heart, allow this mist to expand through the front of your body and fill the southern quarter as far as you can imagine into the horizon in front of you. Visualize the red mist turning into a wall of fire. See the fire moving up to the sky and expanding far and wide, filling the southern horizon in front of you. Visualize a giant red phoenix, the guardian of the Fire Element, rising from the flames.
- Breathe once into the pearl in your Dantian.
- Bring your attention to your kidneys, breathe into your kidneys and imagine a blue/black mist filling them, allow the mist to expand through the back of your body and fill the northern quarter as far and as wide as you can imagine into the horizon behind you. Visualize the blue/black mist turning into a vast deep ocean and expanding far and wide, filling the northern horizon behind you. Visualize a giant black turtle, the guardian of the Water Element, swimming through the waves into the horizon.
- Breathe once into the pearl in your Dantian.
- Bring your attention to your spleen, breathe once into your spleen and imagine a golden yellow mist filling it. Visualize the yellow mist encircling your body; allow it to expand so that it encompasses all the other four elements. Imagine the yellow mist turning into an Earth; see it above you, below you and all around you, embracing all the other elements.
- Breathe once into the pearl in your Dantian.
- Bring your attention to Baihui Du20 and visualize a trap door opening, extend your consciousness up into the heavens and imagine the constellation of the plough or big dipper and the north or pole star. Imagine the energy of the two meeting as a bright white light and then pouring down in a great pillar of light through the heavens, in through the trap door at Du20 and moving powerfully down through your whole body and down through your roots into the Earth. Imagine this white light energy moving through you and washing over you like a great waterfall charging you with universal Qi.
- Bring your attention back to the pearl in your Dantian and breathe into it nine times.
- To finish, rub your palms together until they are hot and put them over your eyes. Circle your eyes behind your palms three times in each direction and then massage your ears and tug them up and down three times. This will help to bring you out of a meditative state and back into day-to-day reality.
- Be as imaginative as you like with this exercise to establish the images that really work for you. After you have practiced it once a day for a fortnight you will be able to do it very quickly in just a few minutes. I suggest you practice it once in the morning and then at any time during the day when you feel you need it.

Relaxing and focusing the mind

'Where your mind goes your Qi follows.' Working with a clear but relaxed and gentle attention is an essential key to giving effective treatments and a skill that generally takes time to develop. The exercises below will help you to learn how to bring your mind and Qi to your hands, increase the sensitivity of your hands and help you to relax, soften and let go enough to allow the healing intelligence of the universe to flow through you and out of your hands.

To begin with, practice for 5 minutes per day for 2 weeks, increase this to 10 minutes for a further 2 weeks and eventually build up to 20 or 30 minutes.

Holding the ball of Qi (Fig. 1.3)

Stand with your feet shoulder width apart and knees slightly bent. Put the tip of your tongue on the roof of your mouth behind your teeth. Lengthen your spine and relax your whole body as much as possible. Imagine a string attached to the back of your wrists and someone lifting your wrists up to the level of Zhongwan Ren12. Turn your wrists so your palms are facing up and your fingers are pointing towards each other. Keep your shoulders relaxed and your elbows away from the sides of your body. Imagine balloons under your arms and your upper

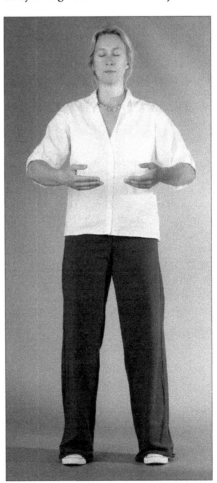

Fig. 1.3 Holding the ball of Qi.

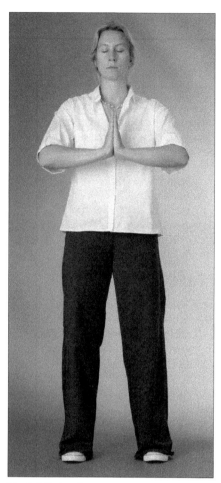

Fig. 1.4 Pericardium prayer.

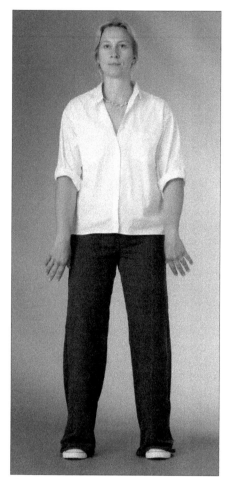

Fig. 1.5 Rattling the bones.

arms resting on them. Close your eyes and bring your attention to your palms. Imagine you are holding a very light paper ball in your hands. Be aware of any sensations that you feel in and around your palms. When your mind wanders, gently bring it back to focusing on your palms.

Pericardium prayer (Fig. 1.4)

Sit comfortably on a chair or stand with your feet flat on the ground and your spine straight. Bring your hands into a prayer position in front of your chest. Put the tip of your tongue on the roof of your mouth behind your teeth. Close your eyes and focus your attention at the place where your Laogong PC8 points meet or where the tips of your middle fingers meet. When your mind wanders, just gently bring your attention softly back.

Cleansing and clearing

After treating a patient and at the end of a clinic day, it is important to take a little time to cleanse and clear your energy field. Between patients this can be achieved quickly in the following way:

1. Dredge your arm channels with Tui fa, imagining that you are drawing out any stagnant pathogenic Qi.
2. Imagine a bucket on the floor in front of you, cross your left hand over your right at the wrists and shake your arms forcefully, shaking any pathogenic or stagnant Qi out of your hands through the Jing Well

points and into the bucket. Do the same with each leg, imagining any sick Qi clearing out through Yongquan KD1.
3. Wash your hands in warm water.

Rattling the bones and coffee press detox

This is a great cleansing and clearing exercise to use at the end of a clinic day and at any time when you are feeling unwell such as when you have a cold.

- Stand with your feet shoulder width apart, knees slightly bent and arms by your sides. Keep everything very loose and relaxed and begin to bounce up and down a little; gradually begin to shake and rattle your whole body (Fig. 1.5). As you shake and rattle your bones imagine any stagnation or sick Qi stirring and loosening up and coming to the surface. Increase the shaking movement until it is quite vigorous. Then come to a sudden stop. Close your eyes and feel the sensation of the sick Qi swirling around. Imagine a bucket on the floor in front of you, inhale deeply drawing the sick Qi up into your mouth, then bend forwards, open your mouth, stick your tongue out and exhale the sick Qi out through your open mouth into the bucket. Repeat this three times.
- Come back to center, standing with your arms by your sides. Inhale and raise your arms up sideways, palms facing upwards until your hands are above your head. As you do this, imagine gathering the

healthy Qi that you need from the world and the universe around you. As you exhale, press your palms down in front of your body from your head to your feet, pressing any remaining sick Qi down into the Earth. Imagine a cafetière of coffee. Everything below your palms is sick Qi being pushed out and everything above your hands is white light Qi coming in from the universe filling you and recharging you. Do this several times until you feel clear. When you have finished, bring your attention to the pearl in your Dantian and breathe into it for a couple of minutes. (Fig. 1.6A–J)

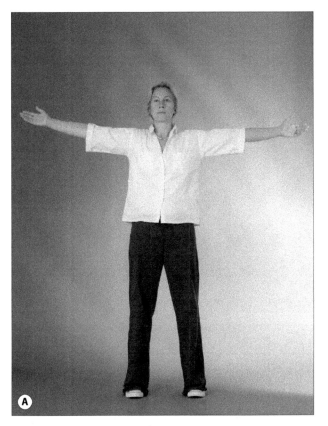

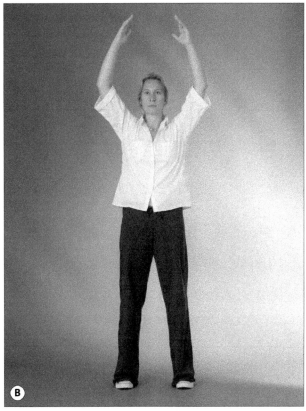

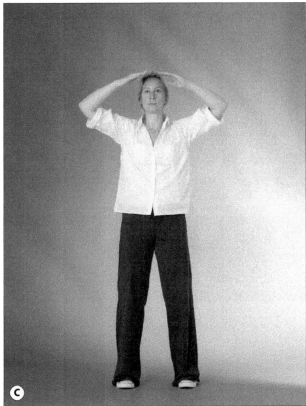

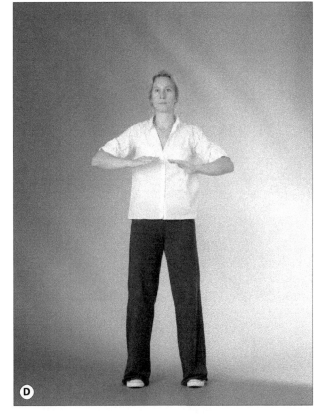

Fig. 1.6A–J Detox sequence.

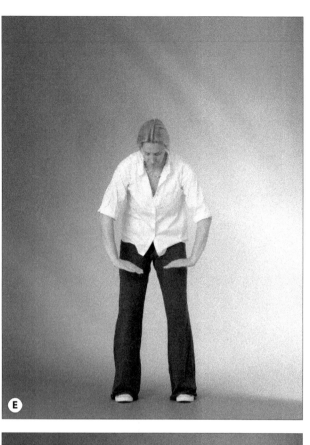

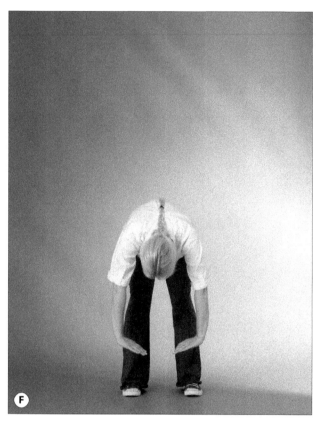

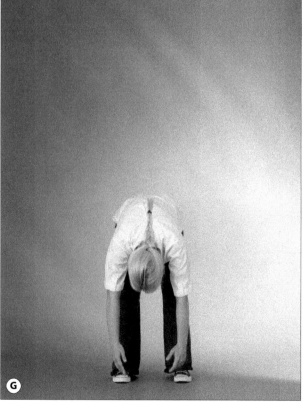

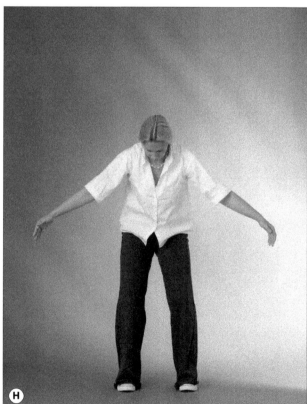

Fig. 1.6A–J *Continued.*

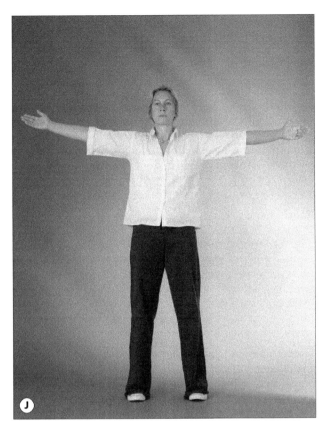

Fig. 1.6A–J *Continued.*

- You can imagine pushing sick Qi out of any level such as your skin, organs, bone marrow and so on.

General health and fitness

As a Tui na practitioner you need to maintain your general health and fitness levels so that you can, if you wish, see several patients a day and practice for many years without burning out. Practice regular Qigong and give time and importance to maintaining your own health. Each person will have different needs: for example, if you lack flexibility then yoga would be a good choice; if you are aware of any postural problems try the Alexander Technique which teaches you how to use your body with the minimum amount of tension and the maximum efficiency. Run, walk, swim or take up whatever works for you and makes you feel good. Eat a regular balanced and varied diet.

Have regular treatments yourself!

Have a Tui na treatment once a month to maintain your health and prevent disharmony. Having treatments is essential to learning; you need to feel and experience the treatment that you are learning to give.

Self-massage

Give yourself Tui na on a regular basis to maintain your health and prevent disease. Self-massage provides a good workout and will strengthen your hands and help you to develop your Tui na techniques.

I suggest that you adapt, simplify and utilize the area foundation routines described in Chapter 7 of this book to create a simple self-massage routine that you can apply before your Qigong practice. Do some work on your head and face, neck and nape, upper limbs, chest and ribs, abdomen and lower limbs.

Yin and Yang styles of practice

Yin and Yang styles of Tui na developed because of the climate and environment that the original practitioners were working in. The Yang style developed in the cold northern parts of China, primarily to deal with Excess Yin and Yang Deficiency. Treatment would frequently be aimed at expelling pathogenic Cold, strengthening Wei Qi, warming Yang, and invigorating and promoting the circulation of Qi and Blood. The Yin style developed in the hot southern parts of China to deal with Excess Yang and Deficient Yin. Treatment would commonly have involved cooling, soothing and calming the patient, sedating Yang and nourishing Yin.

The treatment challenges that we face as 21st century Tui na practitioners in the West are different to those of practitioners working hundreds of years ago in China. It is common to see patients who have both Excess and Deficiency as part of their presenting disharmony. Although both approaches can be applied to a wide range of ailments, each style has its own particular strengths and the potential to affect Qi in different ways.

I believe that it is of great benefit to both ourselves as practitioners and to our patients if we have the ability to work with both approaches. I encourage students to learn, explore and work with both Yin and Yang styles of practice. Some students and practitioners have a natural flair for working with one style or the other and may choose to specialize in working with that style alone. Most, however, integrate the two approaches, find their own middle ground and have the flexibility to be able to move to either end of the Yin–Yang scale, as treatment requires it.

Both styles can be learnt only by working with teachers who are skilled in these approaches, by observing and feeling, and by hands-on practice and experience. Below is an outline of the strengths and effects of the two approaches, and some suggestions for when to use them.

Yang style

Yang style is dynamic and physical. A moderate to strong Yang style is what you will see in the Tui na departments of the TCM hospitals in China. A wide range of basic, compound and coordinated techniques can be employed. The techniques are applied powerfully and vigorously in the analgesic stage of treatment. Points and channels are stimulated strongly until the patient feels 'de qi' sensations such as soreness, numbness and distension. Techniques flow and move rhythmically from one to another, moving, warming, invigorating, exciting, dispersing, dredging and clearing.

Effects
Invigorates Qi, moves Qi and Blood, breaks up stagnation and stasis, disperses accumulations, adhesions and

congestion, warms and strengthens Yang, clears and dredges the channels and collaterals.

When to use Yang style

- When a disease is acute, Excess and Exterior or has strong symptoms; an obvious example of this would be an acute invasion of Wind-Cold
- For channel sinew muscular skeletal problems, to release and relax the channel sinews and break up fibrous adhesions from old injuries
- To release emotional and postural holding patterns from the channel sinews
- To facilitate the movement of joints
- For Bi syndrome, especially Wind-Cold-Damp
- Any problems related to stagnation and stasis of Qi and Blood, e.g. dysmenorrhea
- To strengthen Wei Qi
- Accumulation, congestion and stagnation of Yin pathogens, Damp-Cold and Phlegm
- Warming and strengthening Yang

Yin style

In Yin style there is far less obvious outer physical activity. The practitioner works from a still, very relaxed, centered and grounded place. A smaller range of techniques are employed: these are commonly Mo fa, Tui fa, Rou fa, An fa, Ba shen fa and Yao fa. Techniques are applied gently, slowly and subtly to an area, channel or point for a relatively long period of time. The practitioner directs their attention and Qi into points, channels, bones and organs, to soothe, calm, cool, sedate, slow down, contain and nourish. Space and time are given for the patient's awareness, breath and Qi to come to the area being treated and for changes to take place from within.

Effects

Soothes Qi, regulates Qi, sedates Yang, slows down the movement of Qi, calms the Shen, draws and gathers Qi to a depleted area, nourishes Yin and Blood.

When to use Yin style

- If a disease is chronic, Deficient and Interior, for example Kidney Yin Deficiency with Empty Heat rising manifesting as menopausal syndrome
- If a disease is hidden, deep or 'mysterious' such as myalgic encephalitis (ME), Parkinson's disease
- To nourish Blood and Yin
- To cool Empty Heat
- To aid the healing of old fractures and bone traumas
- To tonify the Zangfu

Other methods commonly applied in Yin style Tui na

Holding and connecting points

For example, to nourish Lung Yin, hold Taiyuan LU9 with the middle finger of one hand and Zhongfu LU1 with the middle finger of your other hand. Direct your Qi and attention down through the points with your treatment intention in mind. Wait for a sensation of warmth, or a slight numbness at the tips of your fingers to occur. This method can be applied to any two points or simply to one point. Use your thumbs or middle fingers. Subtle Rou fa can be added to the holding action.

Tai chi hands

Put your hands either side of the area to be treated, for example around the shoulder joint. Visualize a ball of Qi in the center of the joint and subtly roll the ball of Qi around between your palms inside the joint. If you are working with the organs, you could visualize the color associated with that organ. Give the technique time, and allow space for the patient's breath and Qi to create changes from within.

Holding and pulsing the bones

There are specialist forms of Yin style Tui na, which are very subtle. These practices originated from shamanic medicine, and are essentially forms of Qigong or 'hands on' healing. One example of this is the method of holding and pulsing the bones. This method creates changes in the Qi of the bone, drawing Qi back to places that have been starved for some time and helping to correct the flow of Qi through the channels.

Hold the bone or bones you want to affect between your palms. For example, to affect the sacroiliac joint, put one hand on the patient's sacrum and the other on their ileum. Bring your attention through the skin and muscles, down to the level of the bones. Imagine you are literally holding the bones between your hands. Give time and space to feel that connection and then create a subtle pulsing movement between your hands. Imagine you are energetically pulsing the bones towards each other and then relax and let your hands follow the subtle movements of Qi that occur.

This method is being successfully employed in the early stages of the treatment of Parkinson's disease. Practitioner Janice Walton-Hadlock discovered a link between Parkinson's disease and the retrograde movement of Qi through the Yang Ming and Shao Yang channels caused by traumatic injuries to the bones of the foot and lower leg. For further information about Janice Walton-Hadlock's work on the treatment of Parkinson's disease, see the resources section at the end of the book.

SECTION TWO

Techniques and methods

推拿

CHAPTER **2**

Introduction to Tui na techniques

This section of the book will help you to learn the Tui na techniques that are most commonly applied in the treatment of adults. There are four categories of techniques:

1. Basic techniques
2. Compound techniques
3. Coordinated techniques
4. Passive movements

For each technique, I describe how to practice and apply it, where on the body it can be applied, its therapeutic actions and clinical applications. To help the learning process, you will find a tips for practice box for each technique to remind you of the key points and common pitfalls. Please note that from now on, the English translation for each technique will be given in italic directly after the pin yin name, e.g. Gun fa *rolling*.

As with any practical subject, it is difficult to learn Tui na from a book. To make things as clear as possible, in addition to the accompanying photographs, each technique is also demonstrated in the videos that accompany this book, these are available at www.singingdragon.com/catalogue/book/9781848192690/resources.

What you will need for practice

Fortunately, very little equipment is needed in the practice of Tui na.

Couch

You will need a height-adjustable treatment couch. A hydraulic or electric one is ideal in the long term, but a manually-adjustable one is also fine. I recommend that you keep your couch fairly low so that you can comfortably apply techniques that require pressure.

Chair

You will also need a chair without arms or a stool. Tui na is often applied to patients in a seated position for treatment of areas such as the head, neck, shoulders and upper limb.

Rice bag

The most difficult techniques, Gun fa and Yi zhi chan tui fa, must be practiced and perfected on a rice bag before attempting to apply them to a human being. Striking technique Ji dian fa should also be practiced on the rice bag. As rice bags are not easily available, you can make your own out of strong but soft cotton – nothing too coarse, as you are going to be rolling the back of your hand onto it for several months to come.

The bag should be about 30 cm (12 in) long by 15 cm (6 in) wide and 10 cm (4 in) deep. Fill it with rice so that it is quite firmly packed. There is a story that the old Chinese Tui na teachers would give their students a rice bag after showing them how to practice Gun fa and Yi zhi chan tui fa, and tell them to return when they had ground the rice down to powder through their practice. Only then were they ready to work on a human body!

Tui na sheet/cloth

Unless a massage medium such as an external herbal application is being used, Tui na is generally applied through a sheet or cloth which is wrapped around the patient to create a smooth and even surface to work on. The Tui na sheet should be about the size of a single bed sheet and made of soft cotton, ideally brushed cotton, which is very comfortable to work over.

The patient can be in their underwear with the sheet wrapped around them or they can remain clothed with the sheet used over the top of all the clothes. In China, patients are often treated fully clothed.

Personally I find it more practical on the whole to work with the patient in their underwear so that I can get to the skin easily to apply a massage medium, gua sha, cupping, moxa or acupuncture. Working over a T-shirt and tracksuit bottoms, or the equivalent, is also quite acceptable.

Other equipment

You will also need the following items for the application of ancillary therapies.

For cupping

- Glass cups – I suggest you invest in a selection of sizes, e.g. 4 small, 4 medium and 2 large cups should be adequate
- Forceps
- Surgical spirits
- Cotton wool
- Lighter
- Base oil, such as grape seed, to be applied to the skin before cupping

For moxibustion

- Loose moxa punk
- Moxa sticks
- Moxa box
- Moxa extinguisher
- Closable moxa ashtray
- Akebane sticks
- Gua sha implement – I recommend the horn gua sha sticks – they are easy to use and therapeutically very effective

Basic massage media

- Talc
- Toasted sesame oil
- Red flower oil
- White flower oil
- Woodlock oil
- Essential oil

For more information on external herbal massage media, see Chapter 9.

See the resources section at the end of the book for suppliers of the above items.

How to practice

Practicing Tui na can be physically and energetically demanding. Patience and persistence are what most of the techniques require. The therapeutic qualities of many of the techniques are brought about by performing them for relatively long periods of time so regular daily practice is essential.

At the beginning of Tui na training I suggest that you create a practice regime that consists of 15 minutes Gun fa and Yi zhi chan tui fa practice on the rice bag. Practice of these two techniques strengthens the muscles, tendons and joints in the hands and arms, making the other basic and compound techniques easy to acquire. After a couple of weeks, increase your practice time by 5 minutes each week until you are able to practice for 30 minutes – 15 minutes of Gun fa and 15 minutes of Yi zhi chan tui fa. After about 3 months and if you are feeling confident and comfortable with the techniques on the rice bag, start to practice on your fellow students or colleagues but keep the rice bag practice going as well for the first year of practice. I also suggest that you practice Ji dian fa on the rice bag every day to build up your accuracy and skill.

All the other techniques require much practice on lots of different bodies. One of the best ways to get this experience is to get together with other students to practice and play with the techniques. If this is not possible, then ask as many friends and relatives as possible if you can practice on them. Finally, practice the area foundation routines in Chapter 7 – they will help you to develop the fluidity of moving from one technique to another.

CHAPTER

Basic techniques

Gun fa *rolling*

Unlike techniques such as Rou fa *kneading* and Na fa *grasping* which usually feel pleasant and instinctive to apply, Gun fa (like Yi zhi chan tui fa) initially feels awkward and unnatural to perform. This is one of the hardest techniques to master and it takes time and practice to get it right.

Gun fa can be applied in a very focused way to one particular area such as the shoulder joint, or it can be moved gradually along a channel or section of a channel. It can be accompanied by passive movements of a joint, particularly the neck and shoulder.

It is essential that you learn to do Gun fa with both hands as its therapeutic qualities come about through performing the technique for relatively long periods of time; 20 minutes is quite usual so it is useful to be able to swap hands. The area or side of the body you are working on will also dictate which hand would be best to use.

Gun fa can also be applied with both hands working simultaneously. This is most common when working down the Bladder channel on the back.

How to practice Gun fa

Gun fa must be practiced on a rice bag before attempting to apply it to a human body. It will take about 3–4 months of daily practice to get to grips with it on the rice bag, and a further 6 months to begin to feel really comfortable and competent with the technique.

 Starting position (Fig. 3.1)

- Put your rice bag on a table in front of you and slightly to one side. The table should not be too high; you need to feel that you can relax the weight of your arm down onto the rice bag. If you are practicing with your right hand, place the bag slightly to your right; this will give you enough space to allow your elbow and upper arm to swing freely.
- Stand with your feet shoulder width apart and knees slightly bent, or in a forward lunge posture.
- Place your little finger knuckle onto the rice bag, fingers relaxed and loosely curled. Imagine your knuckle is glued to the spot (some students find it helpful to mark a spot on the bag). The little finger knuckle is the pivotal point and never leaves the spot.

Step one – rolling out (Fig. 3.2)

Initiating the movement from your elbow, rotate your forearm and extend your wrist, rolling the triangular area between your fifth and third knuckles and the head of your ulna onto the rice bag smoothly and evenly. Keep rolling out until your wrist is fully extended, palm facing upwards, fingers extended but relaxed. Your elbow and upper arm should now be out, away from the side of your body.

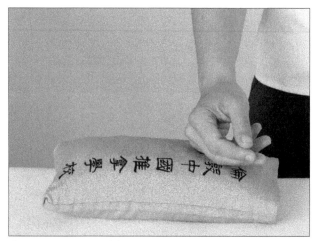

Fig. 3.1 Gun fa *rolling* 滾法: showing how to practice on a rice bag.

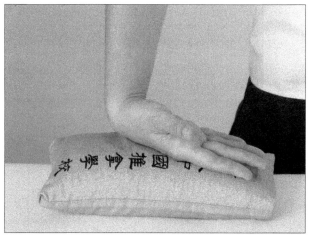

Fig. 3.2 Gun fa *rolling* 滾法: showing how to practice on a rice bag.

Step two – rolling back

Keeping the little finger knuckle glued to the spot, bring your elbow and upper arm back to your side allowing your wrist to straighten and the back of your hand to roll off the rice bag back to the starting position.

Initially, practice for 10 minutes each day, 5 minutes with each hand. Let your dominant hand teach your non-dominant hand. Start slowly and get it technically correct. Apply the natural weight of your arm plus a little more. Do not add too much pressure at the start of practice – just enough to make you feel securely in place. Remember that the rolling movement does not start in your hand. It is your elbow and the extensor muscles of your forearm that propel and power the movement. When observed from behind, the elbow should look like a chicken's wing rhythmically moving back and forth. Think of your hand as a greasy metal ball rolling smoothly with constant even pressure.

Build your practice up to 20 minutes per day, and after 2 or 3 months, your wrist will be more flexible and your muscles stronger. At this stage you can begin to practice on the human body. Ideally, practice on fellow students, colleagues, friends and family and try applying Gun fa to a variety of areas. As you become more competent, gradu-

ally use your body weight to add more pressure to the area you are treating. Build up your speed bit by bit to the optimum 120–160 cycles per minute.

Suggestions for practice on a volunteer

I suggest you start by practicing on the lower back, focusing your technique on one area such as around Shenshu BL23 for several minutes and then gradually moving down the Bladder channel, over the buttock and down the leg to the ankle. Once you have arrived at the ankle, swap hands and work your way back up to the lower back. When using Gun fa to move from one place to another like this, the little finger knuckle acts as a guide focusing the technique along the channel and on any specific points that require attention along the way.

With your volunteer sitting in a chair, apply Gun fa around Fenchi GB21 in a focused manner then try moving from here up to Jianjing GB20. You will need to hold their head with your other hand and gently tilt it away from the side you are working on (Fig. 3.3). This is an example of Gun fa plus passive movement. Repeat on the other side.

Also in the sitting position apply Gun fa to the shoulder joint. Hold the volunteer's arm around the elbow with your other hand, keeping their forearm close to your body. This will help to support their arm properly and keep you in a good position for applying passive movement to the joint. (Fig. 3.4)

If you are working on your volunteer's left shoulder, stand facing their back, hold their arm with your left hand and apply Gun fa all around the posterior aspect of the joint. Standing in a forward lunge and moving from your Dantian, rock forward and back to create some simple passive movement or twist and rotate their arm to expose more of the San Jiao and Small Intestine channels. Then move around to work on the anterior aspect of the joint. Now your left arm applies Gun fa and the right arm the passive movements. From this position, twist and rotate to expose the Lung channel.

Tips for practice

- Relax, close your eyes or look anywhere other than your hand for half the practice time.
- Be as smooth and rounded as you can. There should be no jerky movements.
- Concentrate on your elbow and upper arm moving in and out like a chicken's wing flapping in and out. Or think of squeezing air out of bagpipes that are under your armpit.
- Be consistent in pressure and speed. Start gently and moderately if working on a painful area, gradually building up speed to between 120–160 cycles per minute.
- Your fifth finger knuckle should stay in contact with the area being treated at all times.
- Use music to help you get into a steady rhythm.
- Keep breathing and watch your posture; keep upright and avoid hunching.

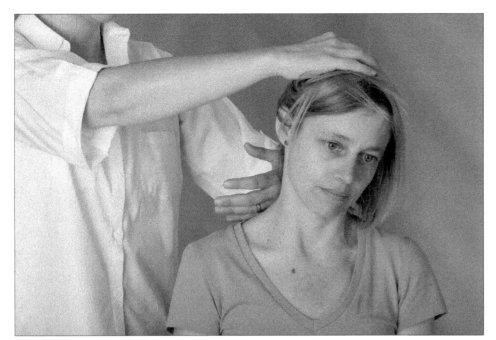

Fig. 3.3 Gun fa *rolling* 滚法: applying to the neck and nape.

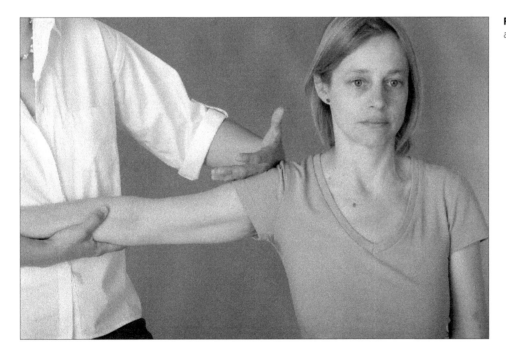

Fig. 3.4 Gun fa *rolling* 滚法: applying to the shoulder joint.

Watch out for the following common mistakes that can develop during the initial months of practice:

1. Incorrect hand positioning
2. Driving the movement from the wrist rather than from the relaxed free movement of the elbow and forearm
3. The technique becomes jerky rather than smooth usually from adding too much pressure too soon
4. The pressure is uneven, usually too strong rolling out and too weak rolling back
5. The technique is too light and superficial rubbing back and forth over the skin surface

Clinical application and therapeutic effects

Where to apply the technique on the body

Gun fa is generally applied to joints and to large muscular areas, shoulders, back, waist, buttocks, hips, arms and legs. It can be used to stimulate points when applied in a very focused manner. It is often used along the course of the channel sinews and the primary meridian pathways. It can also be applied to the abdomen and the pectoral muscles of the chest.

Therapeutic effects

Gun fa has a deep, penetrating and warming effect. It can be used effectively to move through from the adaptive to the analgesic level of treatment. In this case the application starts gently, relatively superficially and at a moderate pace. Gradually over a period of 5–10 minutes it becomes increasingly deeper and more driven, building in pace.

Gun fa dredges the Jingluo, clearing pathogenic Wind, Cold and Damp. It promotes the circulation of Qi and Blood and disperses stasis. It relaxes tendons and muscles, helps to break up adhesions, alleviates pain and muscle spasms, reduces swelling and lubricates joints.

Common uses

- Use Gun fa for any type of Bi syndrome, any channel sinew problems such as muscular pain and stiffness, soft tissue injuries and repetitive strain injury (RSI). Use it for back pain and sciatica, frozen shoulder and tennis elbow.
- Gun fa is an essential technique in the treatment of Wei syndrome including post-stroke sequelae and all forms of paralysis and dysfunction of the motor nerves. Use it for any case that involves numbness and pins and needles in the limbs.
- It is also very effective as part of treatment for abdominal pain with Fullness and distension caused by Qi stagnation.

Yi zhi chan tui fa 一指禅推法
one-finger
meditation pushing technique

Yi zhi chan tui fa is the Tui na practitioner's equivalent of the acupuncturist's needle. It is used for stimulating points along the meridians. A clue to the technique is in its name. Chan means meditation, which suggests prolonged focus and attention in a relaxed manner. Yi zhi chan tui fa is a small, focused and repetitive rocking motion of the thumb, propelled by the wrist and forearm.

Like Gun fa *rolling*, it is a difficult technique to master and feels initially awkward and unnatural to perform. Students often become very frustrated with Yi zhi chan tui fa in the first weeks of practice, when it tends to feel uncomfortable unless you have very flexible wrists. It needs perseverance and lots of practice on the rice bag before beginning to apply it to patients, but with a few months of dedicated practice, Yi zhi chan tui fa can become an incredibly powerful therapeutic tool.

The Yi zhi chan tui fa school or style of Tui na which uses Yi zhi chan tui fa as the main manipulation is one of the most influential schools of thought in the development of Tui na, probably because of its ability to treat at the level of the Zangfu as well as the channels, making it therapeutically wide ranging.

How to practice Yi zhi chan tui fa

It is important to learn to do Yi zhi chan tui fa with both thumbs. Start by practicing on your rice bag for 2–3 minutes a day with each thumb and gradually increase by 2–3 minutes each week until you reach about 20 minutes of practice per day. It can feel particularly awkward and uncomfortable when you first start, but after a few months of regular practice it will become more natural. Practice slowly for the first few weeks then, as you become more familiar and confident with the technique, start to build up your speed. In practice, this technique is applied at 120–160 cycles per minute.

After about 2 months of consistent practice you can start to work on points on fellow students and willing volunteers to develop your technique further and build up your confidence of learning to adapt to different areas of the body.

The technique can be broken down into the following three steps.

Step one – preparation

Mark a spot on your rice bag – this represents a point to be stimulated. Sit with your rice bag on a table in front of you and slightly to the side of your dominant hand. Have both feet flat on the floor, about shoulder width apart.

Place either the tip or pad of the thumb of your dominant hand on the spot. Whether you use the tip or pad depends on your personal anatomy – if your distal thumb joint is very flexible, you will find it easier to use the pad; most people, however, need to use their thumb tip. Keep your thumb perpendicular and curl your fingers into a loose, hollow fist. Do not hold your fingers tightly. Relax your shoulder and imagine your arm is resting on a tennis ball in your armpit. Drop your elbow so that it is lower than your wrist – this is often what makes the technique feel awkward, especially if your forearm extensors are tight and your wrist is not very flexible. Rest your other hand on the rice bag. (Fig. 3.5)

Step two – rocking out

Keeping your thumb 'glued' to the spot, allow the natural weight of your arm to drop into the rice bag. Using the muscles of your forearm, rock your wrist and relaxed fingers away from your body, extending your thumb. (Fig. 3.6)

Step three – rocking in

Flex your forearm muscles and rock your wrist back towards you, bringing your fingers in towards your thumb, which now flexes backwards slightly. If you have a very flexible distal joint then you do not need to flex it backwards; just rock back and forth on the pad of your thumb. (Fig. 3.7)

These steps complete one cycle. Repeat this over and over again to get the flow and rhythm of the movement. As you practice, build up your speed.

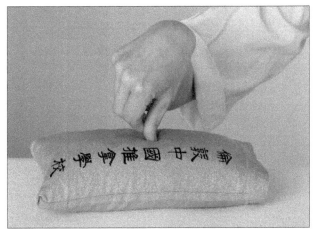

Fig. 3.5 Yi zhi chan tui fa *one-finger meditation* 一指禪推法: practicing on a rice bag, preparation step 1.

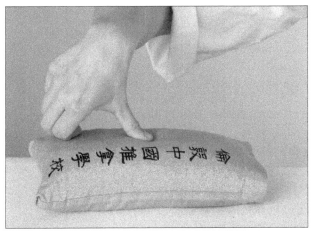

Fig. 3.6 Yi zhi chan tui fa *one-finger meditation* 一指禪推法: practicing on a rice bag, step 2.

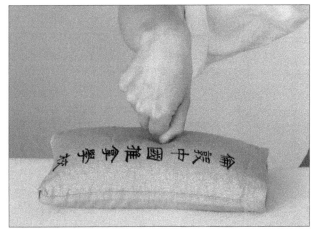

Fig. 3.7 Yi zhi chan tui fa *one-finger meditation* 一指禪推法: practicing on a rice bag, step 3.

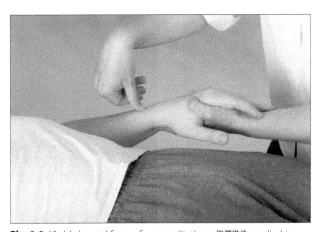

Fig. 3.8 Yi zhi chan tui fa *one-finger meditation* 一指禪推法: applied to a point on the body.

Applying Yi zhi chan tui fa to points (Fig. 3.8)

The focused, rhythmic oscillation of Yi zhi chan tui fa produces a particular vibratory frequency. This frequency creates its therapeutic effect and ability to stimulate the qi and the actions of the points.

To tonify

Apply the technique gently. Propel the movement in the direction of the natural flow of the channel. Visualize Qi coming from the universe and moving through you to the tip of your thumb and into the point. Stimulate the point in this way for about 3–4 minutes or until you feel warmth at the point and the patient feels some sensation such as a mild ache in the local area.

To disperse

Apply strong stimulation by rocking your wrist and thumb powerfully and vigorously. Use the full weight of your arm but do not be tempted to use hard muscular force. Propel the movement against the natural flow of the channel. Stimulate the point for about 1.5 minutes or until the patient feels a strong ache in the local area.

Always keep the treatment principle, your intention, in your heart and mind.

Moving Yi zhi chan tui fa

Yi zhi chan tui fa can also be used along sections of channels or from point to point. It is most commonly used in this way on the face. I use this method on the back down the Bladder channel and along the Huatuojiaji points. The radial edge of the thumb is used rather than the tip.

Clinical application and therapeutic effects

Where to apply the technique on the body

Yi zhi chan tui fa can be applied to all points, along channels and from point to point.

Therapeutic effects

These are wide ranging as Yi zhi chan tui fa stimulates the therapeutic actions of the points. You could, in theory, only use Yi zhi chan tui fa in a treatment. In this way it works like acupuncture in that you decide upon a points prescription that fulfils your treatment principle and then you apply Yi zhi chan tui fa in an even, tonifying or dispersing manner.

Yi zhi chan tui fa activates the circulation of Qi and Blood, and disperses Qi stagnation, Blood stasis and food

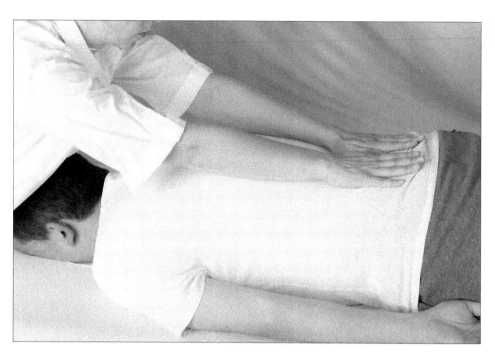

Fig. 3.9 Tui fa *pushing* 推法: two palms on the back.

Tips for practice

- For point stimulation keep your thumb glued to the point at all times. Do not let it wander around off course.
- Make sure your shoulder is relaxed. Do not let it creep up towards your ear. Imagine your arm is resting on a tennis ball in your armpit.
- Keep your elbow lower than your wrist.
- Keep relaxed and get into a rhythm with the movement.
- Use the weight of your arm, not muscular force which will create stagnation.
- Close your eyes or look anywhere other than your hand for at least half of your practice time.
- Focus your mental attention and your energy gently on the tip of your thumb.
- Keep a sense of softness even when dispersing.
- Be patient and persevere.

retention. It is often used to strengthen the Stomach and Spleen and to regulate and harmonize Wei and Ying Qi.

Common uses

You can use Yi zhi chan tui fa as part of your treatment for most disharmonies. It is used to treat both channel problems and Zangfu disharmonies. Some common clinical uses are:

- Headaches
- Insomnia
- Dizziness
- Hypertension
- Abdominal and epigastric pain
- Poor digestion

- Gynecological problems and fertility issues
- Traumatic injury and Bi syndrome

Moving Yi zhi chan tui fa is very useful on the face for sinus problems, and as part of a treatment for facial rejuvenation.

Tui fa *pushing*　　推法

Tui fa is a relatively simple technique to perform. It involves pushing from one place to another, usually along a meridian or part of a meridian. It can be applied over clothes and a Tui na sheet, or directly onto the skin if you want to use an external herbal formula or massage medium. Tui fa can be applied with the thumb, fingers, palm, heel of the palm, knuckles or the elbow. (Fig. 3.9)

Tui fa is often used as an adaptive technique at the start of treatment. It will entice the Qi to move, relax the patient and help you to open up the channels in the limbs and create space for dredging out unwanted pathogenic Qi. In this case the application is brisk and fairly light.

It is also an excellent technique for returning to at various stages in a treatment to clear and dredge the channels of any pathogenic Qi that may have been stirred up. At this stage the application is usually stronger, deeper and more driven.

How to practice Tui fa

Palm Tui fa

Put the whole of your palm and fingers onto the area to be treated and focus your attention on Laogong PC8. Apply a little pressure using the weight of your arm. Push in a straight line forwards along a channel, then immediately pull backwards along the same line. This completes one cycle. The forward pushing should be

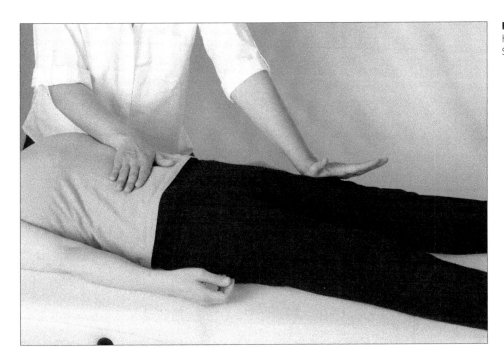

Fig. 3.10 Tui fa *pushing* 推法:
heel of the palm down the
Stomach channel on the thigh.

reasonably strong and penetrating and the backward movement, which is really just a way of keeping in contact with your patient, should be soft and gentle.

Try practicing using both palms on either side of the spine. Stand at the head of your volunteer and focus your Laogong PC8 points on the Bladder meridian. Allow your Qi to gather at your palms by focusing your mind there. Push down the Bladder channel from the top of the shoulders to the buttocks until the whole area feels warm (see Fig. 3.9). Then stand to one side of your volunteer and push with one palm from the buttocks to the end of the little toe. Repeat on the other side.

To add more pressure, try reinforcing the technique by putting one hand on top of the other and applying pressure with the top hand.

Heel of palm Tui fa

Put the heel of your palm on the area to be treated. Extend your wrist and your fingers; the fingers can be closed or slightly separated. Using the heel of the palm gives you a firmer pressure and is useful in areas with larger muscle groups such as the lower back, hips and thighs. (Fig. 3.10)

Thumb Tui fa

Use either the pad of your thumb or the radial side. Tuck your fingers into the palm or rest them on the body. This method is useful on the face, head and neck and for tonifying points, particularly Back Shu points, in which case you apply the technique gently and with many repetitions: 100–300. (Fig. 3.11)

Finger Tui fa

Use the pads of your index and middle fingers or index, middle and ring fingers to push along sections of meridians. This is commonly used on the neck, chest, forearm and lower leg.

Elbow Tui fa

This is most commonly used on the back, down either side of the spine to stimulate the Huatuojiaji points. Apply a suitable massage medium first then put the tip of your elbow just to one side of the spine. With the palm of your other hand, guide and support the elbow; to do this make an 'L' shape between your thumb and index finger and cradle the elbow there. This makes the patient feel more comfortable and supported. Apply pressure with your elbow and push, sliding slowly down the back with your other palm behind. (Fig. 3.12)

Knuckle Tui fa

Using one or both hands, make a loose fist and push with the middle sections of your knuckles. I use this frequently on the soles of the feet to stimulate Yongquan KD1. It can be applied to most muscle groups, especially of the back, arms and legs.

Tips for practice

- Think of planing wood or ironing.
- When using palm Tui fa keep your attention on Laogong PC8. Line your Laogong up with the channel you are working on.
- Make it rhythmic, consistent and smooth.
- Enjoy it; it should feel good to you as well as the patient.

Clinical application and therapeutic effects

Where to apply the technique on the body

Tui fa is extremely versatile and can be applied all over the body.

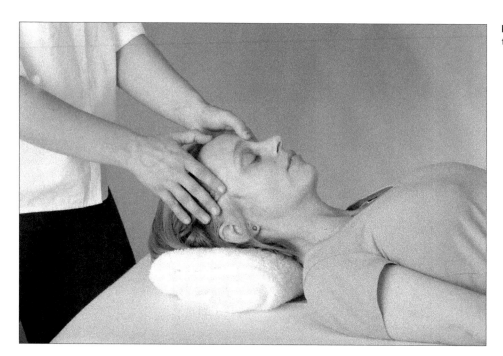

Fig. 3.11 Tui fa *pushing* 推法: thumbs on the face.

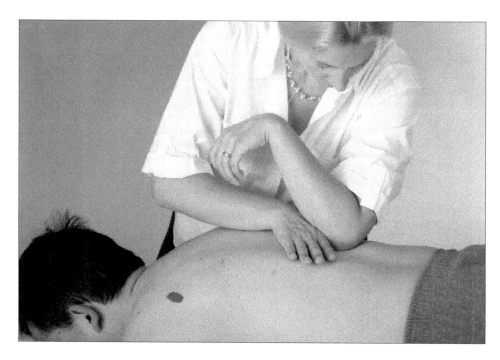

Fig. 3.12 Tui fa *pushing* 推法: elbow on the back.

Thumb and finger pushing are used mainly on the face, head, neck, nape and chest. Palms are used on the back, hips, belly, ribs, chest, arms and legs. The heel of the palm is used on the chest, belly, back, arms and legs. The elbow is used on the back, hips and thighs. The knuckles are used on the back, arms, legs and soles of the feet.

Therapeutic effects

This depends on the area of the body that it is applied to and how it is applied. Generally Tui fa opens and warms the meridians, dredges the meridians, moves Qi and Blood, relaxes the muscles and sinews, relieves pain,

clears the head, promotes circulation of Qi in the chest and aids respiration, strengthens the Stomach and Spleen, improves digestion and harmonizes the Middle Jiao.

Common uses

Tui fa can be used during most treatments for all sorts of complaints. Use it to start treatment in the adaptive stage and come back to it if you want to dredge a channel. Common indications for its use are:

* Headaches
* Dizziness
* Anxiety

- Hypertension
- Insomnia
- Cough
- Asthma
- Oppressive feeling in the chest
- Digestive problems
- Abdominal distension
- Stiff neck
- Muscular spasm
- Bi syndrome
- Backache

Rou fa *kneading*

Rou fa is one of the most versatile and flexible Tui na techniques. You can use it anywhere on the body and can apply it with your thumb, middle finger, all four fingers plus your thumb, your whole palm, heel of your palm, major or minor thenar eminence. It can also be performed using the forearm or elbow for stronger, more vigorous stimulation. Rou fa is the root technique for four compound techniques (see p. 66) and because of its flexibility is often used as part of the coordinated techniques (see p. 73).

Rou fa has wide-ranging therapeutic qualities depending on which form is used and how it is applied. For example, you can use your thumb and middle finger to stimulate points. You can use your palm on the abdomen to tonify the Stomach and Spleen and harmonize the Middle Jiao. If you apply Rou fa with your elbow to Huantiao GB30 and then with your forearm across Ganshu BL18 and Danshu BL19, it will help Excess Liver disharmonies such as Liver-Fire, Liver-Yang rising and Liver-Qi stagnation. You can use Rou fa in one area or point or you can move along a channel to dredge it of obstructions, relax the muscles and invigorate the flow of Qi and Blood.

How to practice Rou fa

The warmth that is generated from the soft repetitive, relatively slow circular kneading creates Rou fa's therapeutic effects. The warmth generated when the technique is correctly applied moves down into the deep tissue layers. The rule with Rou fa, whichever part of your body you are using, is to move the underlying muscles and not the skin. It is important to keep your hand and wrist as well as your Qi and breath soft. Rou fa should feel both gentle and deep.

Example of working with your palm on the belly

Put your palm on your patient's belly and focus your Laogong PC8 on your patient's Zhongwan Ren12. Center and ground yourself and bring your breath, mind and Qi to your palm. Allow the weight of your arm plus a little additional pressure to drop down into your palm. Begin to knead circularly in a clockwise direction keeping your palm fixed and moving the underlying muscles (Fig. 3.13). Do not rub over the skin surface. Keep softness in your hand and wrist. Start slowly and gradually increase the speed to about 100 circles a minute. Knead until you feel the area become very warm. Repeat this over Qihai Ren6.

Now put the ulnar side of your forearm across your patient's navel to stimulate Tianshu ST25, Daheng SP15 and Huangshu KD16. You will need to adopt a low posture with your knees bent. Keep your shoulder relaxed and begin to knead with your forearm in a clockwise direction. (Fig. 3.14)

Example of working on points

Sit or stand depending on which part of the body you are working on and what feels most comfortable.

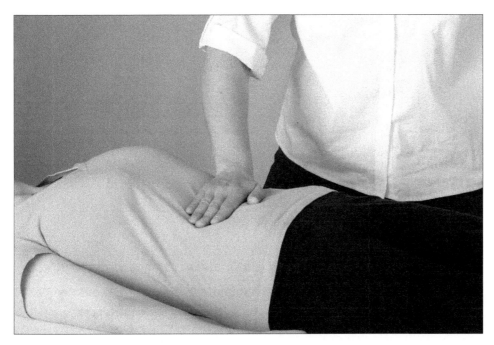

Fig. 3.13 Rou fa *kneading* 揉法: palm on the belly.

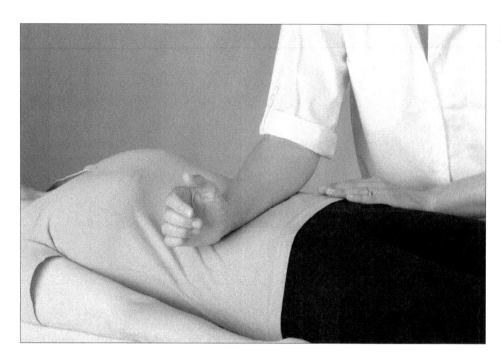

Fig. 3.14 Rou fa *kneading* 揉法: forearm on the belly.

Using your thumb

Choose a point to work on. Put the pad of your thumb onto the point and let your fingers relax naturally onto your patient's body. Allow the weight of your arm to relax into the point and begin to knead gently and slowly.

If you want to tonify, continue to use gentle kneading in a clockwise direction. Keep your intention gently in mind and continue for a minimum of 3 minutes. To disperse, apply Rou fa in an anti-clockwise direction for a shorter period of time, about 1.5 minutes. Add more pressure by using your body weight and increase the speed of the technique until you are doing roughly 140–160 circles per minute.

Using your middle finger

Place the pad or tip of your middle finger onto the selected point. For support hold the distal joint between your index finger at the top and your thumb at the back. Use the natural weight of your arm. Knead the point in a continuous circular motion as above.

Example of various forms of Rou fa working down the back and lower limb

With your patient lying down prone, stand to their right-hand side. Apply Rou fa using your whole palm at first and then the heel of your palm. Work down the right-hand side of the Bladder channel kneading the underlying muscles in generous circles. Knead several times in one spot to make the area warm, and then move down a little and repeat, working down the channel gradually from the shoulder to the sacrum. To create stronger stimulation and to move muscles that are very bulky or tight, use your other hand on top for support. Do this three times with the whole palm, then three times using the heel of your palm. Repeat on the left.

Now apply Rou fa to your patient's sacrum and sacroiliac area using the heel of your palm and the major and

minor thenar areas. Swap between these methods using whichever part of your hand fits most comfortably. Try using both hands together either side of the sacrum and around the hips. (Fig. 3.15)

Now using the tip of your elbow, work deeply and briskly into major points around the buttocks such as Baohuang BL53, Zhibian BL54 and Chengfu BL36. When you work with your elbow, keep your wrist and hand relaxed. For support and for your patient's comfort, cradle your elbow in the 'L' shape formed between the index finger and abducted thumb of your other hand and let that hand join your elbow in the kneading. (Fig. 3.16)

Using the heel and thenar areas of your hand, apply Rou fa from Zhibian BL54 down to Chengjin BL56. Work down the channel three times increasing the speed and strength gradually. Finally, apply Rou fa with your thumb from Chengjin BL56 all the way down the channel to Zhiyin BL67, paying attention to major points along the way. Repeat on the left side.

Tips for practice

- Always move the underlying muscles and do not skim over the surface of the skin.
- Rou fa should feel soft and comfortable, deep and penetrating.
- You can stay in one place or move from one place to another, e.g. over the whole muscle group or along the course of a channel.
- Start slowly and gently, gradually increasing your pressure and speed.

Clinical application and therapeutic effects

Where to apply the technique on the body

Rou fa can be used anywhere on the body. Thumb and finger Rou fa is mainly used on points. The major thenar

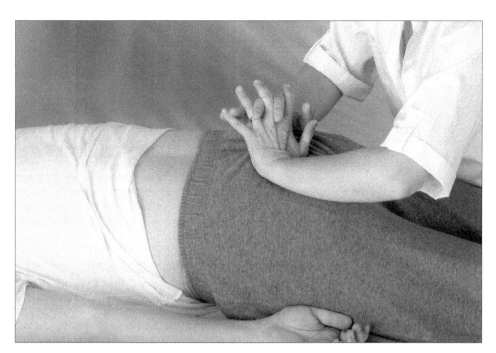

Fig. 3.15 Rou fa *kneading* 揉法: heels of palms around the sacro-illiac area.

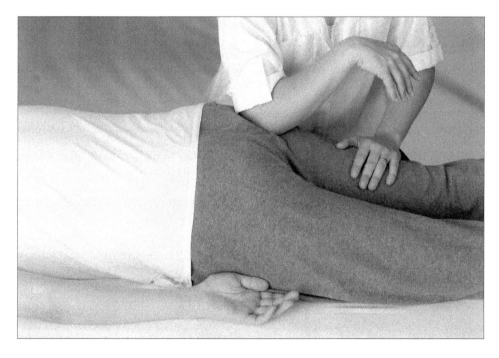

Fig. 3.16 Rou fa *kneading* 揉法: elbow on the buttocks.

area and the thumbs and middle fingers are used for the face and head. The heel of the palm, whole palm, thenar areas and forearm are used for the back, hips, legs and shoulders. The heel of the palm, thenar areas, fingers and thumbs are used for the arms. The whole palm, forearm and fingers or thumb are used on the abdomen. Elbow Rou fa is used mainly on the large muscular areas of the back, hips and thighs.

Therapeutic effects

As stated above the therapeutic effects of Rou fa are very wide ranging depending on the method of Rou fa and the area of the body being treated. Rou fa stimulates the

actions of the points, invigorates and regulates the flow of Qi and Blood, reduces swelling, relaxes the muscles and relieves spasm, stops pain, dredges the channels, expels Wind and Cold, opens the chest, strengthens the Stomach and Spleen, harmonizes the Middle Jiao and calms the mind. If you apply brisk and strong elbow and forearm Rou fa it will subdue rising Liver-Yang, clear Liver-Heat and generally soothe, cool and regulate the Liver.

Common uses

In practice Rou fa is probably the most commonly used Tui na technique and I would be surprised to see a treatment that did not include some version of Rou fa. The following are some common indications for Rou fa:

- Headaches and migraine
- Dizziness
- Insomnia
- Constipation
- Diarrhea
- Epigastric pain and distension
- Hypochondriac pain
- Oppressive feeling in the chest
- Menstrual pain
- Muscular pain
- Numbness
- Stiffness and spasm
- Bi syndrome
- Backache
- Soft tissue injuries
- Sprains
- Hemiplegia
- Stress
- Anxiety and depression

An fa *pressing*

Chinese massage was originally called 'An wu' or 'An mo' which gives us a strong indication of the therapeutic importance of An fa. It is one of the most ancient of all techniques. Shiatsu developed from the ancient roots of 'An wu' and uses the therapeutic qualities of An fa as a major part of treatment to great effect.

In terms of the three levels of treatment, An fa is applied at the heart of a treatment in the middle or an-algesic stage. It is one of the most versatile techniques and can be used anywhere on the body to stimulate points,

joints and the primary channels. It is commonly blended with Rou fa *kneading* technique.

How to practice An fa

The application of An fa requires sensitivity, awareness and a relaxed mental focus from the practitioner. The thumbs are used to stimulate most points. The tips of the middle fingers can also be used; this is useful for points on the head, chest and rib area. Knuckles provide stronger stimulation, particularly for the back and for larger muscle groups. The palm, heel of the palm, major or minor thenar muscles are used for larger areas such as the back, buttocks, legs and belly.

Example of An fa using the thumb
(Fig. 3.17)

Choose a point to be stimulated and bring the pad or tip of your dominant thumb to the point. If you are using the tip of your thumb, curl your fingers into a loose fist and support your thumb's distal joint against your index finger. If you are using the pad of your thumb, keep your fingers relaxed naturally onto your patient's body.

Relax your shoulders. Check that you are grounded and centered and that your breath is moving freely. Initially, just be aware of the gentle contact you have with your patient as you just hold the point. Be aware of the actions of the point and your intention. You will feel the point warming and opening at this level.

Now, using your Qi and breath, start to push into the point. Use the weight of your hand and arm at first and then gradually apply more pressure using your body weight, not your muscular strength. Always start gently, gradually increasing the pressure to the desired level. The depth of the pressure will depend upon several factors, such as the location of the point, your intention in stimu-

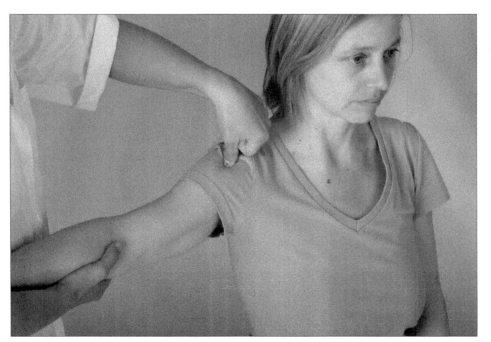

Fig. 3.17 An fa *pressing* 按法: tip of the thumb in the shoulder joint.

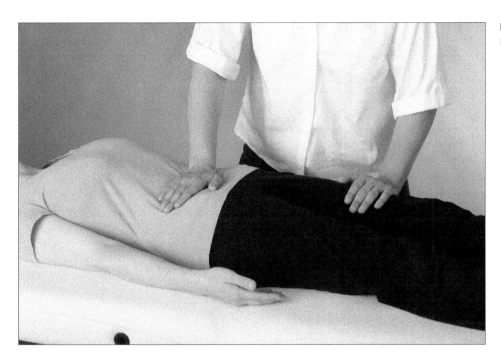

Fig. 3.18 An fa *pressing* 按法: palm on the belly.

lating it, whether you are tonifying or dispersing, taking a Yin or Yang approach and so on.

Your thumb will become warm or a little numb after about a minute; this is a sign that the Qi is moving and the point is open and activated. The patient will probably feel an aching sensation at or around the point. Generally pressure is maintained for about 3 minutes at a point; of course this is only an average and the time can be decreased or increased according to the patient and treatment required. You can use your non-dominant thumb on top of your working thumb to reinforce the pressure and to relieve any strain on your thumb joints.

Another method of applying An fa is to press intermittently and rhythmically. This is useful to disperse and to work along small sections of the channels. Apply An fa in the same way with your middle finger or knuckles.

Example of An fa using the palm and heel of the palm

With your patient lying down supine, place your palm on their belly. Relax, ground and center yourself. Send your breath into your Laogong PC8 point. Starting at the level of the Dantian, apply pressure gradually as above (Fig. 3.18). Work with your patient's breath. As they breathe in release your pressure and as they breathe out apply pressure. Work gradually and slowly in clockwise circles encouraging them to deepen their breath as you work. After several circles have been completed begin to work down their Stomach channel with the heel of your palm from Tianshu ST25 to Jiexi ST41. Do this three times on each side. Keep in contact with your patient at all times as you move along the course of the channel – just release your pressure and slide along to the next place.

When you are working on the limbs and back, remember to use your body weight to give you deeper pressure (Fig. 3.19). You can reinforce the pressure by using your other hand on top.

If your patient is very Deficient, you can hold gentle to moderate pressure for up to 5 minutes. If you want to move stagnation, only pause briefly before releasing the pressure.

Tips for practice

- Relax, check that you are grounded and centered and that your breath is moving freely.
- Use your Qi and breath as you start to push into the point.
- Use body weight, not muscular strength, for additional pressure.
- Take your time and do not 'bash' at it.
- You can reinforce the pressure by using your other hand or thumb on top.
- Do not break contact as you move along the course of a channel.
- Enjoy it. The more relaxed you are, the better it will be.

Clinical application and therapeutic effects

Where to apply the technique on the body

An fa can be used anywhere on the body to stimulate points and channels.

Therapeutic effects

These are wide and varied because, as with the other point-stimulating techniques, the nature and spirit of the individual points are awakened. The effects:

- Slow, steady, gentle to moderate pressure for longer periods of time (over 3 minutes) will tonify, support and strengthen the channels, vital substances and Zangfu, calm the Shen, dispel anxiety and relax and strengthen muscles and tendons.

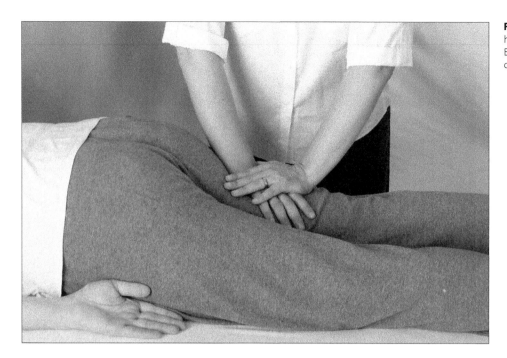

Fig. 3.19 An fa *pressing* 按法: heel of the palm down the Bladder channel along the back of the leg.

- Deep An fa held for 3 or more minutes will relieve pain, spasm and stasis and help to adjust and realign joints.
- Quick, rhythmic pressing and releasing will move and disperse stagnant Qi and Blood.
- Applied along the course of a channel using moderate pace and pressure, An fa will warm the channels and regulate and harmonize the flow of Qi and Blood and the functions of the Zangfu.
- Applied on the abdomen, An fa will aid digestion and remove retention of food.

Common uses

An fa can be used in any treatment plan for any problem. Some common indications for its use are:

- Insomnia
- Anxiety
- Headaches
- Digestive disorders
- Respiratory problems
- Menstrual disorders
- Fertility problems
- General muscular aches
- Pains and stiffness
- Trauma
- Bi syndrome
- Joint misalignment

Ya fa *suppressing* 壓法

Ya fa is really a stronger, more intense, version of An fa. It belongs at the analgesic or second level of treatment. It is applied with the tip of the elbow, the forearm and, on occasion, the knees or heels if you are working at floor level. It is used where very strong, persistent stimulation is required on large muscular areas and points that are deep, such as Huantiao GB30.

In practice I use Ya fa a great deal, and not just because it gives my thumbs a break and requires no physical effort on my part, although this is a great bonus. I have found that persistent strong elbow suppression followed by intermittent suppressing and releasing can really help to shift deeply held tension and stasis so commonly found in the Bladder and Gallbladder channel sinews in the back, buttocks and legs.

How to practice Ya fa

Example of applying Ya fa with your elbow
(Fig. 3.20)

Choose a point on the Gallbladder or Bladder channel to stimulate. Adopt a grounded and centered stance. Place the tip of your elbow onto the point. For stability and for your patient's comfort, use the support of your other hand. Do this by abducting your thumb so that you have formed an 'L' shape between thumb and index finger and nestle your elbow into this shape.

Now begin to lean into the point using your body weight. Lean in very gradually, slowly increasing the pressure by allowing your body weight to drop more into the point. Keep your awareness at your elbow; you may be surprised at just how sensitive an elbow can be! Be aware of what is happening under your elbow: are you feeling your patient's muscles hardening against your pressure? If so you need to back off and ask them to work with you by bringing their breath and attention to the point. The sensation felt by your patient should be quite a strong ache. Often patients will feel Qi moving along the channel. Encourage them to let you know what they are feeling so that you can follow this during the treatment.

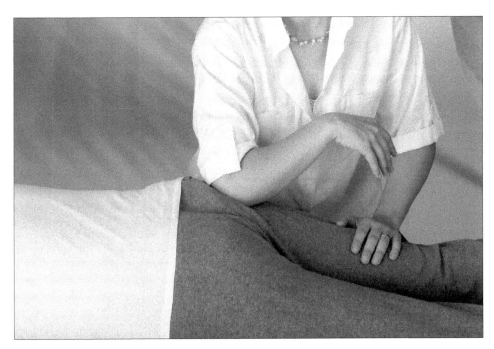

Fig. 3.20 Ya fa *suppressing* 壓法: elbow in Huantiao GB30.

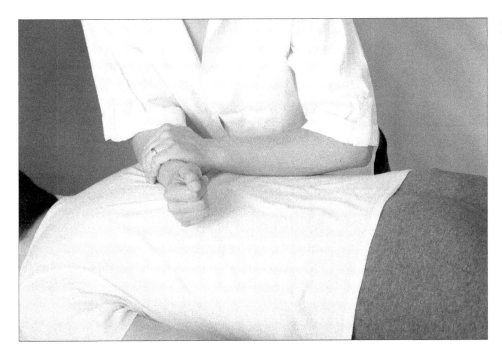

Fig. 3.21 Ya fa *suppressing* 壓法: forearm on the back.

Pause for about 3 minutes or until you feel the point become very warm and have a sense of opening or releasing under your elbow, then gradually release the pressure. You can then suppress and release the point briskly and rhythmically to disperse what has been released. For even deeper suppression, reinforce by using your other hand to hold the fist of your working arm.

Example using your forearm (Fig. 3.21)

With your patient lying prone, start from a grounded, centered posture. Choose an area to treat on your patient's back such as across Ganshu BL18 and Hunmen BL47, the inner and outer Back Shu points for the Liver. Put the ulnar side of your forearm across the spine and both sets of points. Make a loose fist. Suppress slowly and gradually using your body weight. For further reinforcement you can use pressure on top from your other hand. Hold the suppression strongly for about 3 minutes. In addition to the suppression you can rock rhythmically from time to time for further stimulation and release.

Clinical application and therapeutic effects

Where to apply the technique on the body

Ya fa is applied to large muscle groups and deep points and is used mainly on the back, buttocks and legs.

Tips for practice

- Do not be frightened of leaning your body weight onto your patient. It will only hurt if you hold back and tense up. Keep relaxed.
- Lean in very slowly, gradually and smoothly.
- For very deep Ya fa, reinforce by using your other hand on top.
- Keep your attention at your elbow tip in elbow Ya fa and feel for the warmth and changes that occur.
- If your patient is tensing up, back off and help them to work with their breath.

Therapeutic effects

Ya fa removes obstructions from the channels, relaxes spasm, relieves pain, moves stagnant Qi and Blood, expels Wind, disperses Cold, drains Damp from channels, dredges the channels and subdues rising Liver-Yang.

Common uses

- You can use Ya fa as part of your treatment for back pain including Wind-Cold-Damp Bi syndrome and sciatica.
- Use it for stimulating points on the back such as the Huatuojiaji and Back Shu points.
- Use it when the Bladder and Gallbladder channel sinews in the leg feel Full and congested and tender on pressure.
- Use forearm Ya fa over Liver, Stomach and Spleen Back Shu points to harmonize the Middle Jiao, soothe and sedate the Liver and descend Liver-Yang in cases of hypochondriac pain, digestive disturbance, epigastric pain, belching, dizziness, headache and migraine.
- Work in the Yang channels of the legs in areas where you find Fullness and tenderness.
- You can also use Ya fa in the treatment of emotional stress and depression. Ya fa helps to release the stagnation of held emotions that can get locked into the tissues.

Mo fa *round rubbing*

Mo fa is one of the most ancient and probably the most instinctive of all Tui na techniques. An mo was the ancient name for medicinal massage. When someone injured themselves they would literally be rubbed better. As the healing properties of the natural environment were discovered, injuries would be treated by rubbing with herbal preparations – this became known as Gao mo.

Mo fa is soothing, relaxing and comforting to receive and to give. It is generally applied by using the palm of one hand. In digestive or gynecological problems with underlying Deficiency, Mo fa is applied to the belly with the palms joined; this is often referred to as tai chi Mo fa. When applied to the head, the palm and the pads of the fingers are used. This method is sometimes affectionately termed stroking and caressing the head.

How to practice Mo fa

One palm Mo fa

Stand or sit to perform Mo fa, whichever feels most comfortable. If standing, have your knees slightly bent and feet 1.5 × shoulder width apart. Ground and center yourself, and lengthen through your spine. Let your breath and Qi soften. Focus on your intention, then put your dominant hand onto your patient's body.

Keeping your entire palm and fingers in contact with their body, begin to rub in a circular motion. Keep a gentle focus on Laogong PC8 – this will help Qi to gather there and improve the therapeutic effects of the technique. No downward pressure should be applied, just the natural weight of your hand. Make the movement as smooth, relaxed and even as you can. Keep your wrist soft and flexible. The pace is around 100–120 circles per minute. To regulate and harmonize the Middle Jiao and the Intestines, apply Mo fa to the abdomen clockwise 36 times then anti-clockwise 36 times.

I frequently use this method on the belly to tonify and warm the Stomach and Spleen, harmonize the Middle Jiao, regulate the Intestines and calm the Shen in patients with irritable bowel syndrome (IBS). I also use it around the Kidney Back Shu points and Mingmen Du4 to tonify the Kidneys in patients with problems such as lower backache, fertility issues and depression.

This method of Mo fa can also be applied using the major or minor thenar eminence or the heel of the palm. In practice it is often a case of adapting to the individual patient, the area of the body you are treating and what feels most comfortable.

Tai chi Mo fa – using joined palms

Sit or stand, as described above. Form an 'L' shape between your index fingers and thumbs by abducting your thumbs, then overlap one hand on top of the other by interlocking the two 'L' shapes. Put your joined palms onto your patient's belly, keep your shoulders, elbows and wrists open and relaxed, and begin to rub in a circular motion as you did when using a single palm. (Fig. 3.22)

Tai chi Mo fa is used mainly on the belly and applied in a clockwise direction for strengthening, tonifying and warming. It is most effective when you focus the technique, your attention and Qi around a particular point such as Guanyuan Ren4 or Qihai Ren6.

Mo fa using palm and fingers

If your patient has long hair then you will need to apply the technique over your Tui na cloth. With your patient seated, stand either in front or behind them. Starting from the left side of the forehead, round rub with your palm and finger pads working gradually backwards towards the posterior hairline gently and softly. Then move from the center of the forehead over the crown down to the posterior hairline. Then do exactly the same on the right side. Repeat the round rubbing, gradually increasing the speed of the technique until the head feels warm. (Fig. 3.23)

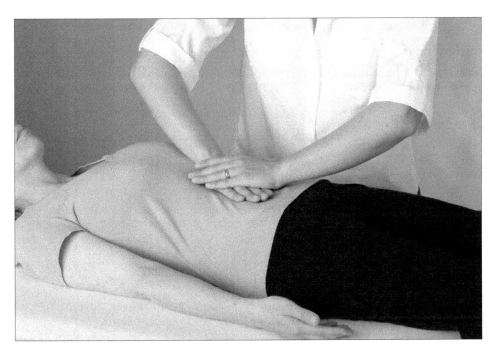

Fig. 3.22 Tai chi Mo fa *round rubbing* 太極摩法: on the abdomen.

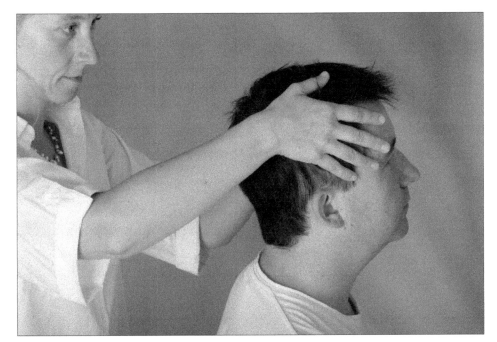

Fig. 3.23 Mo fa *round rubbing* 摩法: on the head.

Mo fa using fingers

Use the pad of your middle finger to apply Mo fa to points. This method is very useful on the face. I like it for opening points and evoking the Qi. It works well before holding and connecting points. You can also use the pads of the middle and index or middle, index and ring fingers to the same effect. Just adapt to what feels most comfortable.

Tips for practice

- Be as relaxed, fluid, smooth and circular as possible.
- Let your wrist soften; let yourself soften.
- Find the rhythm of the movement.
- Bring your attention and therefore your Qi to your palms or fingers.
- Think of polishing something very precious.

Clinical application and therapeutic effects

Where to apply the technique on the body

Mo fa is commonly applied to the chest, ribs, belly, lower back and head. It can also be applied to points using the fingers.

Therapeutic effects

When applied to the abdomen, chest and hypochondria, Mo fa warms and harmonizes the Middle Jiao, strengthens the Stomach and Spleen, improves the digestion, regulates the Intestines, removes food stagnation, soothes the Liver, moves Qi stagnation, disperses Cold and relieves abdominal swelling.

When applied to the head, it expels Wind and disperses Cold and calms the Shen. When applied to the lower back, it tonifies the Kidneys, and strengthens and warms Mingmen.

Apply Mo fa slowly to tonify and strengthen, and briskly to move and clear. When working on the belly, move in a clockwise direction for constipation to increase peristalsis, to remove retention of food and to move stasis. Move anti-clockwise for diarrhea. To tonify Spleen-Qi, you can make small anti-clockwise circles within a large clockwise circle.

Common uses

Mo fa is particularly useful as an adaptive, tonifying and harmonizing technique. Use it for:

- Digestive disorders like IBS, colitis, constipation and diarrhea, epigastric, abdominal, hypochondriac pain and distension and oppressive feelings in the chest
- Menstrual and fertility problems to move Qi and Blood and warm the Lower Jiao and Kidneys
- Headaches, insomnia, shock, anxiety and depression

Ma fa wiping

Ma fa, like Tui fa, is one of the easier techniques to acquire. It is a gentle, brisk technique used mainly on the face, head and neck to calm the mind and bring Qi and Blood to the sense organs, thereby improving their functions. It could theoretically be used anywhere on the body. I use it on the chest frequently and as a dispersing technique after applying deep An fa, An rou fa or Ya fa. It is applied using the pad of one or both thumbs simultaneously.

How to practice Ma fa

You can stand or sit to perform Ma fa, whichever feels most comfortable. Remember to keep your spine straight, your shoulders relaxed and center your breathing in your Dantian. Put the pad of your thumb or pads of both thumbs onto the area you want to treat, relaxing your fingers onto your patient's body. Some students have a tendency to stick their fingers out away from the patient. This creates tension, blocks the flow of Qi and feels a bit strange from the patient's point of view.

Wipe back and forth in a relaxed and brisk fashion in small lines up and down the area you are treating. Be gentle, but not superficial – imagine you are wiping a dirty mark off the skin. The speed of this technique is generally about 100–120 per minute.

Example using one thumb

With your patient lying prone or seated and their neck straight, stand to their left-hand side. Using the pad of your right thumb, wipe back and forth over the Bladder channel sinew of the neck on the left-hand side. Work gradually up and down from Tianzhu BL10 down to the nape. Relax your fingers down onto the right side of your patient's neck and let them move naturally. Repeat this a few times then try doing it on the other side using your left thumb. (Fig. 3.24)

Example using two thumbs

Stand or sit at the head of your patient. Put both thumb tips touching in the center of the forehead at the level of Yin tang, relaxing your fingers down at the sides of the head and holding lightly to steady yourself. Wipe with both thumbs back and forth from the center of the forehead towards the temples and back again. Work in lines all the way up the forehead to the hairline and then back down again. Repeat this 3–4 times.

Tips for practice

- Keep your spine straight and your shoulders relaxed.
- Be gentle, even and rhythmic.
- Do not be too superficial with Ma fa. Avoid floating on the surface of the skin.
- Talcum power is a useful medium to apply with this technique, especially if the patient's skin is quite dry.
- Let your fingers relax onto your patient's body; it will be more comfortable for them and you.

Clinical application and therapeutic effects

Where to apply the technique on the body

The technique can be applied anywhere but most commonly to the face, head, neck and nape. I find it useful on the chest, ribs and the spine between vertebrae.

Therapeutic effects

Ma fa calms the Shen, clears the head, improves the eyesight and brings Qi to the sense organs. It disperses congestion and stagnation, soothes pain, relaxes the channel sinews and aids the circulation of Qi and Blood.

Common uses

Use Ma fa as part of treatment for:

- Anxiety
- Depression
- Sinusitis
- Allergic rhinitis
- Common cold

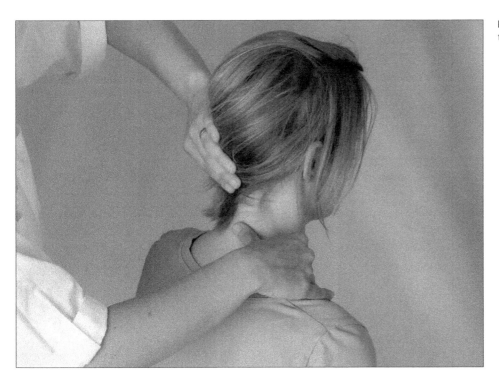

Fig. 3.24 Ma fa *wiping* 抹法: one thumb on the neck.

- Cough
- Asthma
- Headaches
- Facial paralysis
- Dizziness
- Stiff neck
- Myopia
- Insomnia
- Hypertension

It can be used generally for aches and pains to disperse stagnation.

Na fa *grasping*

Na fa is one of the most versatile and frequently used Tui na techniques. As the root technique for at least seven compound techniques, its flexibility in practice is invaluable. In this section I will explain how to apply the basic root technique, leaving the compound versions to the next chapter.

Basic Na fa can be applied in three ways: with the pads of your thumb, index and middle finger; with the pads of your thumb and all four fingers (Fig. 3.25); or with your whole hand (Fig. 3.26). For larger muscular areas such as the buttocks and thighs you can use both hands together.

Na fa is a good technique for self-massage so try it on yourself. You could work on both major points and along the channel sinews in your arms and legs.

How to practice Na fa

Na fa is generally performed from a standing position. Give yourself a solid, grounded base to work from by standing with your feet 1.5 × shoulder width apart and your knees slightly bent.

Example of Na fa working on the upper limb

With your patient lying down supine, support their left arm with your left hand. Begin by grasping the Large Intestine channel sinew at the insertion of the deltoid muscle around Jianyu LI15. Grip and squeeze the muscle between the pads of your thumb and fingers, lift it up away from the underlying bones, then release the muscle. Continue grasping at LI15 for a minute or two until the area becomes warm. Begin slowly and gently, gradually increasing the pace and strength you apply as the area warms up.

Now start to move the Na fa down along the Large Intestine channel sinew, working gradually and paying extra attention to any areas that feel either particularly Full and Stagnant or Empty and Weak. Na fa should be rhythmic and firm but not rough or hard. In the upper arm you could try using your whole hand instead of thumb and fingers. This method gives a stronger stimulation and can be very useful on bulky muscles. To apply whole hand Na fa, grip and squeeze the muscles between the heel of your palm and your fingers.

When you arrive at Quchi LI11, swap back to using your thumb and fingers and grasp LI11 and Chize LU5 until warm before continuing to work gradually down the forearm to the wrist, hand and index finger. Linger a little at the Yangxi LI5/Taiyuan LU9 area at the wrist and again at Hegu LI4.

Clinical application and therapeutic effects

Where to apply the technique on the body

Na fa can be applied to the face, neck and shoulders, upper and lower limbs, back, buttocks and abdomen.

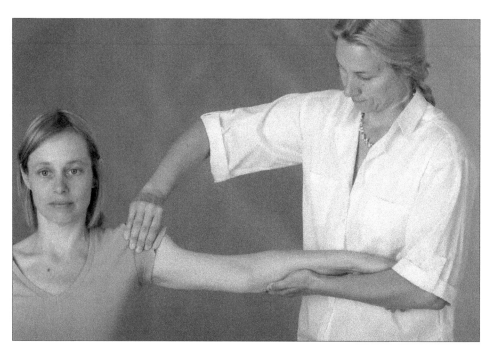

Fig. 3.25 Na fa *grasping* 拿法: thumb and fingers.

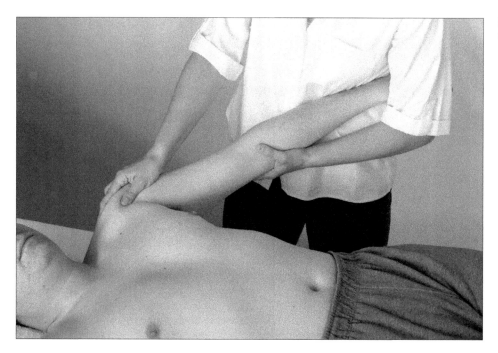

Fig. 3.26 Na fa *grasping* 拿法: the whole hand.

Tips for practice

- Use the pads of your fingers, not your fingertips, and avoid digging your nails into the skin.
- Grip, squeeze and release.
- You can use both hands together for larger muscle groups or larger patients.
- Be firm and rhythmic but not rough and hard.
- Think about warming and softening the area you are working.

Therapeutic effects

Na fa relaxes muscles and tendons, relieves muscle spasm and pain, dredges the channels, expels Wind and dissipates Cold, and promotes circulation of Qi and Blood.

Depending on how it is performed, Na fa can be applied during any of the three levels of treatment. However, it is at its most useful in the analgesic and dissipative stages of treatment. For example, I use Na fa repeatedly in one area to activate major points, to bring Qi and Blood to places that are Empty and undernourished and to break up and dissipate stubborn areas of

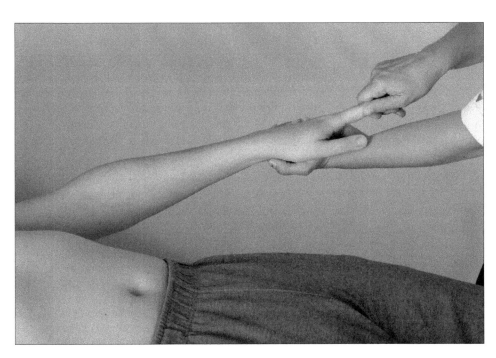

Fig. 3.27 Nian fa *holding twisting*
捻法: to the fingers.

stagnant and congested Qi. Used along the course of a channel sinew, Na fa is great for dredging stirred up stagnation and pathogenic Qi.

Common uses

Because of its versatility, Na fa can be included in most treatments for most problems in some shape or form. It is used to activate major points, bring Qi to Empty areas, clear obstructions, or to dredge the channels. Indications for its use are:

- Channel sinew and joint problems
- Lower backache
- Injuries such as sprains
- Numbness and hemiplegia
- Common cold and hay fever
- Sinusitis
- Headaches
- Stiff neck
- Dizziness
- Poor eyesight

Nian fa *holding twisting* 捻法

Nian fa is applied to the fingers and toes. It is applied with the thumb and index finger or thumb, index and middle finger, depending on what feels most comfortable to you. I use Nian fa during treatment to help to dredge and clear stagnant Qi and pathogenic factors out of the channels as well as for local treatment of the fingers and toes.

How to practice Nian fa

Hold your patient's finger between your thumb and index finger. Hold the digit firmly and twist and rub briskly, moving the underlying joints and muscles. Do not work superficially. Work gradually from the root to the tip of the finger if you are clearing, or remain at one particular joint for a while if there is a local problem. Work each finger several times. Use the same principles if working on the toes.

It is important to dredge right the way through the channels to the extremities and out. The Well points where the polarity of Yin and Yang changes are important doorways for clearing obstructions at the sinew meridian level. (Fig. 3.27)

Tips for practice

- Keep your fingers pliable and relaxed.
- Imagine you are polishing a coin between your thumb and fingers.
- Be firm and work quickly.
- Work each finger several times.
- Coordinate the twisting evenly between your thumb and finger.

Clinical application and therapeutic effects

Where to apply the technique on the body

Apply the technique to the fingers and toes.

Therapeutic effects

Nian fa eases swelling and opens the joints of the fingers and toes. It alleviates pain and numbness, relaxes the muscles and tendons, promotes Qi and Blood circulation locally and through the entire limb or channel. It dredges stagnating obstructions from the channels.

Common uses

Nian fa is used in the treatment of:

- Bi syndrome

- Sprains
- Swelling
- Numbness and pain in the fingers and toes
- Trigger finger and thumb
- Raynaud's disease

It is used as a supplementary technique for most muscular skeletal problems of the limbs, cervical spondylopathy, paralysis and numbness of the extremities.

Ji dian fa
finger striking (also called dotting and pointing) 擊點法

Ji dian fa is the main technique used in the digital striking school of Tui na, which developed from the traditional 'wushu' martial arts. You need strong fingers and arms to perform the heavier versions of Ji dian fa, so if you would like to develop this technique and style of practice you will need to do plenty of Shaolin Qigong and other upper body strengthening exercises.

Ji dian fa is a dissipative technique. In fact, heavy striking is probably the most dissipative Tui na technique that can be applied. The reverberation it creates affects the deepest tissue layers of the body, breaking up and moving stubborn obstructions. Ji dian fa has been used for centuries in China with great success to treat various types of paralysis, Wei syndrome and stubborn or difficult cases of Bi syndrome such as rheumatoid arthritis. It is applied to points, joints and along channels.

How to practice Ji dian fa

Ji dian fa can be applied in the following ways:

- **Single-finger striking.** Strike a point using the tip of your middle finger which is supported by holding the distal joint between your index finger and thumb.
- **Three-finger striking.** Strike points, joints and channels with the tips of your thumb, index and middle fingers, which are held together and kept level.
- **Five-finger striking.** Strike points, joints and channels with the tips of all four fingers and your thumb held together and level.

There are two methods of application: the first is known as 'single' or 'even' striking and the second as 'rhythmic' striking.

In single or even striking the rhythm of the striking is even and the intensity of each strike is the same. This method is generally performed at 2–3 strikes per second.

Rhythmic striking uses a pattern of weak strikes that are light and fast, and strong strikes which are heavy and slow. There are four different possibilities, each with its own pattern of rhythm:

1. One weak strike followed by two strong strikes
2. Two weak strikes followed by two strong strikes
3. Three weak strikes followed by two strong strikes
4. Five weak strikes followed by two strong strikes

Initial rice bag practice is essential. Mark a spot on your rice bag to represent a point to be stimulated. Start by practicing light, even striking using your middle finger, aiming to maintain accuracy and an even rhythm. Sit or stand in a relaxed grounded posture. Relax your shoulder and drop your elbow so that it is lower than your wrist. Put the tip of your middle finger onto the point and hold the distal joint of your middle finger between your thumb and index finger. Light striking comes from the wrist; extend your wrist and raise your hand and then, using gravity, let your hand drop and your finger strike the point. (Fig. 3.28)

Practice the same method using three fingers and then five fingers. Practice with both hands; it is useful in practice to be able to apply Ji dian fa with either hand.

After a week of regular practice on the rice bag, begin to introduce moderate-strength striking. You can sit or stand for this depending on what feels most comfortable. Moderate striking comes from the elbow; keeping your shoulder relaxed, lift your hand, wrist and forearm from the elbow, then allow the weight of your forearm, wrist and hand to drop down and your fingers to strike the point. In all methods of Ji dian fa, your fingers should feel like they are bouncing off the point. You could imagine your fingers as a rubber hammer on a spring. (Fig. 3.29)

After another week of regular practice, introduce a little strong striking into your practice routine. Strong striking comes from the shoulder joint; lift your whole arm up from your shoulder, your hand will come up to your head or above your head, then drop the weight of your whole arm down onto the point. Keep relaxed and flexible in your joints; if you stiffen up or hold your breath and Qi, it will be very uncomfortable to receive. Think of Qi coming from your Dantian and through your arm into your fingers. (Fig. 3.30)

When you feel confident with the light, moderate and heavy versions of single, even striking, begin to practice the four different versions of rhythmic striking. Practice on your rice bag and on your own arms and legs to get a feel for it. As your confidence, strength and ability grow, begin to work on your fellow students and willing colleagues. Work on different points and joints with different methods.

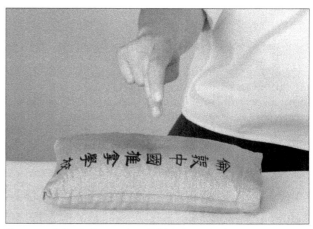

Fig. 3.28 Ji dian fa *finger striking* 擊點法: light single-finger striking on the rice bag.

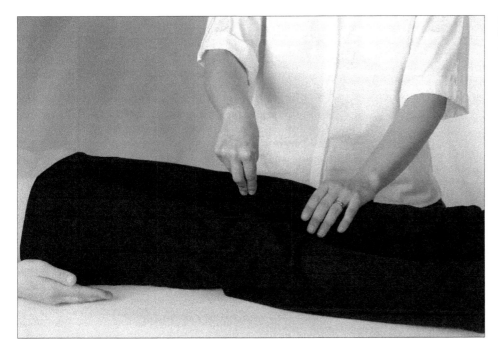

Fig. 3.29 Ji dian fa *finger striking* 擊點法: moderate three-finger striking on the thigh.

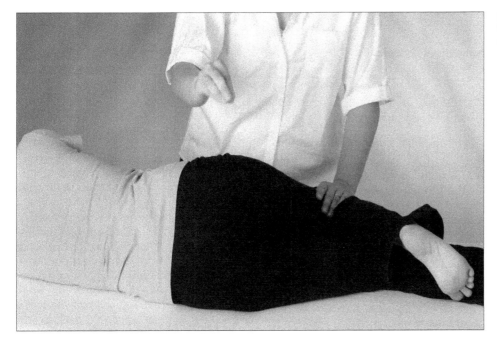

Fig. 3.30 Ji dian fa *finger striking* 擊點法: heavy five-finger striking on Huantiao GB30.

Tips for practice

- Imagine your fingers as a rubber hammer on a spring bouncing off the body.
- Keep relaxed and let gravity do the work.
- Build up strength and speed gradually.
- Focus your mental attention and Qi on your finger tips.
- Breathe evenly and do not hold your breath. Let your breath and Qi move from your Dantian through your arm and down to your fingers.

Clinical application and therapeutic effects

Where to apply the technique on the body

Ji dian fa can be applied to all points, joints and along channels.

Therapeutic effects

Ji dian fa dissipates and clears all pathogenic factors. It clears Heat, quells Fire, expels Wind, disperses Cold and resolves Damp and Phlegm. It activates, dissipates and moves stagnant obstructed Qi and Blood stasis and dredges the channels and collaterals of these obstructions. It relaxes tendons and muscles, relieves muscle spasm, helps the tissues to regenerate, stops pain and opens the joints.

It is used to activate the functions of the points, to harmonize Ying and Wei Qi, strengthen Kidney-Yang and regulate the functions of the Zangfu.

Common uses

Ji dian fa is famous for its treatment of atrophy, painful obstruction and paralysis. Its uses are as follows:

- Use it as part of treatment for Wei syndromes such as multiple sclerosis, poliomyelitis and myasthenia gravis.
- Use it for treatment of Bi syndromes including very difficult cases such as rheumatoid arthritis.
- It is an essential technique to include in all cases of numbness and paralysis from Wind-Stroke hemiplegia to traumatic paraplegia.
- Use it for any type of joint and muscle stiffness and on the Huatuojiaji points as part of treatment for prolapsed lumbar disc.
- Use on head points and distal points according to the disharmony as part of treatment for Shi and mixed Shi and Xu patterns of insomnia, dementia and mental–emotional problems such as anxiety, depression and neurosis.
- Ji dian fa is useful in the treatment of convulsions to help to clear pathogenic Wind, Fire and Phlegm and to descend Qi.

In practice use only light digital striking or slow, soft, rhythmic striking for Xu conditions, weak and elderly patients, children and women during their period or just post-menstrually if Blood Xu, and in the first 6 months after birth.

In cases of one-sided paralysis, atrophy and stubborn cases of Bi syndrome, treat only the strong healthy side of the body with moderate to heavy single and even or rhythmic striking. The dynamic shaking wave that is created by the heavier forms of Ji dian fa resonates through to the affected side, clearing pathogenic factors and moving the obstructed Qi and Blood. In time the obstructed channels begin to open up and the healthy circulation of Qi and Blood is restored.

Medium striking is used a lot today in the West. It has a strong therapeutic effect on deep muscles and is effective for harmonizing the Wei and Ying Qi and dredging meridians. It can be used for Shi conditions and mixed Shi and Xu conditions.

Heavy striking should not be used in the initial stages of treatment. For the first 3–4 treatments start with light striking and gradually increase to a medium striking force. If the patient is accepting this well then gradually continue to increase the force of your striking little by little until you are able to work more heavily. Generally, heavy striking is applied to young, strong adults and to patients with Shi conditions, although there are cases today in a modern Western practice when you have a mixed Shi and Xu condition such as multiple sclerosis (MS) and the Excess must be cleared before tonification. In these cases you can also gradually work towards applying heavy striking if the patient can accept it.

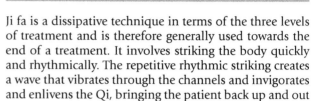

Ji fa is a dissipative technique in terms of the three levels of treatment and is therefore generally used towards the end of a treatment. It involves striking the body quickly and rhythmically. The repetitive rhythmic striking creates a wave that vibrates through the channels and invigorates and enlivens the Qi, bringing the patient back up and out of the analgesic phase of treatment.

It can be applied in several ways, but most commonly with the ulnar edge of the palms working either alternately or with the palms joined together. In practice it is particularly useful for helping to eliminate Phlegm from the Lungs and Damp from the channels.

How to practice Ji fa

The key to applying Ji fa is rhythm and relaxation and a loose flexible wrist.

Example using the ulnar edge of the palms

Although Ji fa can be applied with a single hand it is most commonly applied with both hands working alternately. Stand in a low, stable posture at the head of your patient who is lying prone or seated. Put the ulnar edge or the minor thenar area of both palms either side of your patient's spine. Extend your fingers, keeping your fingers and hands relaxed and your wrists soft and flexible. Start to chop gently either side of your patient's spine using your hands alternately. (Fig. 3.31)

The movement comes from your elbows and wrists, so the more elastic and loose they are the better. If you stiffen up, the technique will become harsh, heavy and uncomfortable to receive. This method of Ji fa is dynamic, but should feel comfortable and pleasant to receive. Imagine your hands are a pair of drumsticks and let them bounce off your patient's body. Keep relaxed and get into a rhythm. Begin gently, at a moderate pace and gradually build up your speed until it is as brisk as you can make it without losing your rhythm and coordination. Work up and down either side of your patient's spine to about the level of their waist and back to the shoulders. Now stand to one side of your patient and work gradually down their back, over the buttocks and down the backs of their legs. Lighten up around the backs of the knees and use more vigor around the buttocks and thighs. Work up and down three times and repeat on the other side.

With joined palms

Join your hands together, palms and fingers touching and cross your thumbs over each other to keep them in place. As above, the movement comes from your elbows and loose wrists. When done correctly, this method produces a sound a bit like slapping down a wet fish! With your patient seated, try applying it to the top of their shoulders and upper back. (Fig. 3.32)

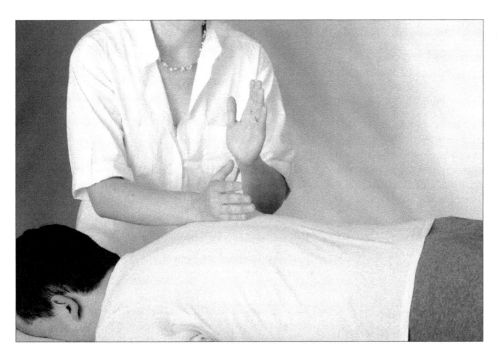

Fig. 3.31 Ji fa *chopping* 擊法: with alternating hands on the back.

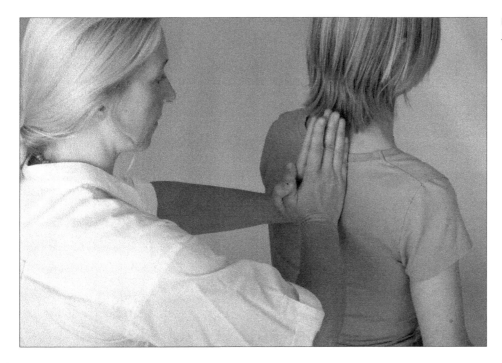

Fig. 3.32 Ji fa *chopping* 擊法: joined palms on the shoulders.

Other alternative methods

Heel of the hand

Apply with wrist extended backwards about 45 degrees, your fingers held together and your thumb abducted.

Center of the palm

Keeping your fingers together and thumb abducted, stretch and arc your palm. This method is generally applied to the vertex of the head.

Tips for practice

- Rhythm and loose wrists are the keys to this technique.
- Whichever method you are using, your hands should feel as if they are bouncing off the body like drumsticks.
- Keep your hands working briskly and lightly; do not let them become heavy and harsh.
- Try practicing to music with a strong beat.
- Ji fa is fun; relax and enjoy it!

Clinical application and therapeutic effects

Where to apply the technique on the body

Ji fa can be applied to the back, buttocks, arms, legs, chest, abdomen, head and shoulders.

Therapeutic effects

Ji fa opens and relieves the chest and eliminates Phlegm when applied to the chest, back and upper limbs. It relaxes tendons and muscles, stimulates and invigorates the flow of Qi and Blood, dissipates stagnation of Qi and stasis of Blood, dredges the channels and eases pain.

Common uses

- Use Ji fa for respiratory problems with Phlegm such as coughs, difficulty breathing, asthma and an oppressive feeling in the chest.
- Use it to invigorate the patient's Qi if they are tired and sluggish due to stagnation and/or Damp.
- Use it as part of treatment for Liver-Qi stagnation leading to flatulence and abdominal distension.
- Use it for Wind-Damp Bi syndrome, hemiplegia, muscular spasm, lower backache, sprain of the lumbar muscles, stiffness and aching of the back, shoulders and limbs.

Pai fa *patting/knocking*

Pai fa is a striking technique used generally at the end dissipative stages of treatment. It is applied with either a cupped palm or a loose fist, using the knuckles, the back or lateral side of the hand. Pai fa is a very useful technique for Phlegm and Damp conditions. I use it a lot in the clinic for clearing Phlegm from the chest and to dredge and clear Phlegm and Damp from the channels.

How to practice Pai fa

Pai fa is usually performed at a moderate speed of about 120 knocks per minute. The exception to the rule is when you are applying it for lighter, more general dissipation with the cupped palm of both hands working alternately along a channel. Otherwise, its pace is not rushed. This gives time in between each knock for the depth and resonance of Pai fa to be felt and its own signature vibration to be created. Allow your hand or loose fist to drop naturally onto the body then bounce back up.

Using a loose fist

This method can be applied in three ways:

1. Using the back of your hand
2. Using the ulnar edge of your hand
3. Using your knuckles

Curl your fingers and thumb into a loose fist. Keep your shoulder relaxed and your elbow and wrist flexible. Pai fa involves the natural lifting and dropping of your loose fist onto your patient's body. Imagine your fist as a rubber beater bouncing off the muscles, knocking softly without any force. Apply Pai fa at a moderate speed keeping your mind and Qi soft as well as your hand and wrist.

If you are using either the back of your hand or your knuckles you can use both fists alternately and rhythmically. The ulnar edge of the hand is generally applied to the vertex of the head using one hand only. (Figs 3.33 and 3.34)

Using a cupped palm

To apply Pai fa with your palm, all your fingers and thumb must be touching. Create a hollow or cupped palm. Leading with a soft flexible wrist, raise your palm

Fig. 3.33 Pai fa *patting/knocking* 拍法: on the back using the back of the hand.

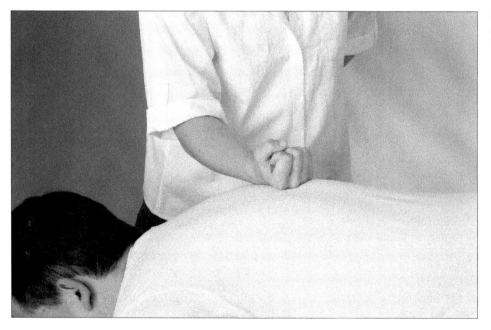

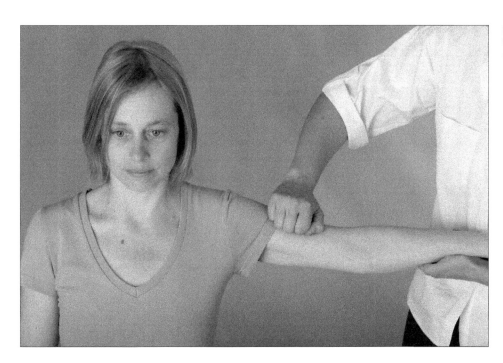

Fig. 3.34 Pai fa *patting/knocking*
拍法: with the knuckles on the
upper limb.

a few inches off your patient's body and then allow it to drop.

Let your hand bounce up and down off your patient's body. Do not use any muscular strength or force. Think of playing a drum like a conga. If you have got it right, your palm will make a hollow, low sound as it strikes the body. If you hear a high slapping sound, it is not right and your palm is probably too flat. (Fig. 3.35)

Tips for practice

- Keep your wrist very pliable – do not stiffen up.
- Do not rush it. Work at a moderate pace, in a relaxed manner.
- Let your palm or fist bounce naturally off the body. Do not be heavy handed.
- Keep your mind and Qi quiet and soft.
- In palm knocking, keep your fingers together and palms cupped and listen for the low hollow sound.
- In fist knocking, keep your fist loose. Do not clench it tightly.
- Knock 3–10 times on any one area.
- Knuckle knocking is like knocking on a door.

Clinical application and therapeutic effects

Where to apply the technique on the body

Pai fa can be used on the back, hips, shoulders, upper and lower limbs, abdomen, ribs and head:

- The cupped palm method can be applied to the shoulders, the abdomen and ribs, the back, hips and legs. It is frequently used over the lower lumbar area and sacrum at the end of a treatment and with both hands working alternately along the course of a channel.

- The ulnar edge of the fist is applied mainly to the vertex of the head.
- The knuckles can be used on the back, around joints and on the arms and legs.
- The back of the hand can be applied to the back and shoulders and also to the arms and legs.

Therapeutic effects

Pai fa relaxes the muscles and tendons, relieving muscle spasms and aching pain. It activates the movement of Qi and Blood and will help in the treatment of Blood stasis. Use Pai fa for conditions that involve Phlegm and Damp. It opens the chest, aids breathing and is very effective for clearing Phlegm from the chest and for dredging the channels of Damp Heat. Applied to the abdomen it can be used as part of treatment to regulate the Stomach and Intestines. Pai fa calms the mind, quells Fire and clears Heat.

Common uses

- Pai fa can be used as part of treatment for headaches and dizziness that are due to either Excess conditions like Liver Fire/Wind or Yang rising, Phlegm and retention of food or mixed Excess and Deficiency such as Liver-Blood Xu/Yin Xu with Yang rising or Spleen Qi Xu and accumulated Dampness. Apply to the vertex and to relevant channels, the back and/or abdomen depending on the condition.
- Pai fa is very useful for coughs with retention of Phlegm, difficulty breathing and an oppressive feeling in the chest; apply to the back, ribs and relevant channels.
- Use Pai fa for nausea, vomiting and digestive problems with a Damp or Damp-Heat component, and for Blood stasis.
- Use it for joint pain from Bi syndrome, especially the Hot and Damp types, and for lower backache.

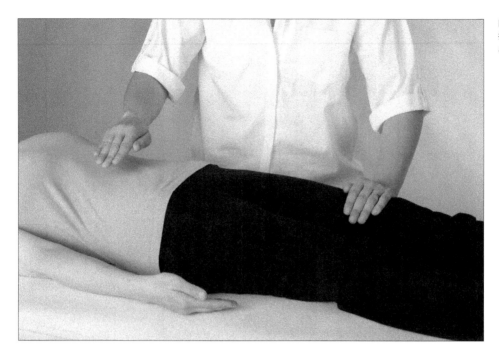

Zhen fa *vibrating*   振法

Zhen fa is a demanding technique for the practitioner to apply and can be a frustrating technique for a student to master. Zhen fa requires you to transmit a high-frequency, up-and-down vibration that penetrates deep into the body. Shaolin Neigong Qigong practice is essential for the development of Zhen fa, as it requires strong, dynamic internal Qi and the ability to draw that Qi from the Dantian to the hand or fingers to create the vibration.

Zhen fa can be used to stimulate any of the points. Finger vibration applied to the head, face and chest points has a tranquilizing effect and will help to calm the Shen when a patient is stressed and anxious. Therapeutically versatile, Zhen fa can be used to relax, calm and warm, to clear Excess, move Blood stasis and break up adhesions. My colleague uses this powerful version of Zhen fa a great deal in his practice to successfully break up adhesions from old trauma. I find palm Zhen fa on the abdomen very effective as part of treatment for digestive disorders and gynecological problems that are caused by either Cold, food and Qi stagnation or Blood stasis.

How to practice Zhen fa

Practice on your rice bag to start with. As the vibration begins to develop, try practicing palm Zhen fa on top of a half-full glass of water – you will see the water moving if you are vibrating correctly. This method of practicing will prevent you at this stage from applying too much downward pressure and will help you to assess how even and constant your Zhen fa is becoming. (Fig. 3.36)

Stand in a grounded and centered posture, with feet shoulder width apart, spine straight and knees slightly bent. Put the palm of your dominant hand onto your rice

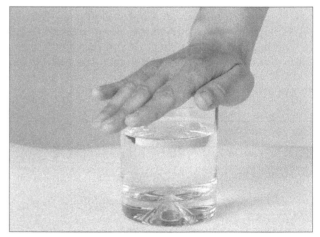

Fig. 3.36 Zhen fa *vibrating* 振法: practicing on a glass of water.

bag. Bring your mental attention down into your Dantian. Allow your breath to drop into your belly and imagine your Qi gathering there. Visualize a pearl in your Dantian; breathe into the pearl and imagine it becoming brighter and more beautiful with each breath. Give yourself time to do this.

Imagine your dominant arm is a hollow tube and internally direct your Qi from the pearl in your Dantian up through your body and then down your arm to the palm of your hand.

Zhen fa requires both relaxation and tension. To produce the vibration, you need to create some tension in your forearm muscles but you must stay as relaxed as possible or the Qi will get stuck on the way and there will be no vibration. Be very aware of your breathing and do not, at any time, hold your breath. This is very important; if you hold your breath when performing Zhen fa, it will have a draining effect on your Qi over time.

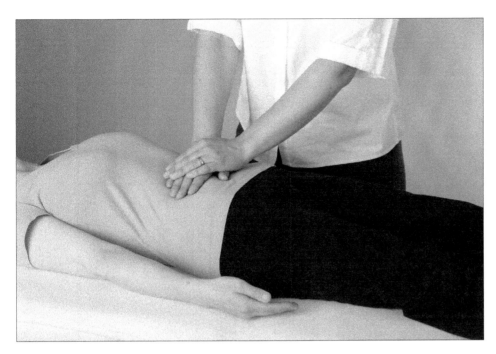

Fig. 3.37 Zhen fa *vibrating* 振法: palm on the abdomen.

Relax your shoulder and keep directing your Qi with your mind from the pearl to your palm. Keep this relaxed tension in your forearm muscles and this will allow a quivering vibration to be created. The vibration is up and down and the frequency is fast.

Practice in short bursts to start with – a little each day. Try after practicing Shaolin Neigong Qigong and you will notice a difference. Build up your practice until you can sustain Zhen fa comfortably for 2–3 minutes. Then begin to apply it to your fellow students and colleagues. To be therapeutically effective you will need to be able to sustain Zhen fa for at least 3–5 minutes.

Zhen fa can be applied in the following ways:

- With the palm of your hand. This method is mainly applied to the abdomen, lower back and sacrum. When using palm Zhen fa, direct your Laogong PC6 over a point on your patient's abdomen or back such as Qihai Ren6. Create contact between the points, imagining your Laogong as a doorway for the vibrating Qi to exit, and direct it into your patient through the point you have connected with. You can apply the weight of your other hand on top for support and a little more pressure. (Fig. 3.37)
- With your middle finger with the distal joint supported by your index finger at the front and your thumb at the back. This method is used to stimulate points. (Fig. 3.38)
- With your middle and index fingers together (sword fingers). This method can also be used to stimulate points and to break up adhesions and masses such as fibroids.
- With your middle finger and thumb. Use this method to stimulate two points at once; this is particularly useful at joints, e.g. you can stimulate Quchi LI11 and Chize LU5 together or Yinlingquan SP9 and Yanglingquan GB34. (Fig. 3.39)

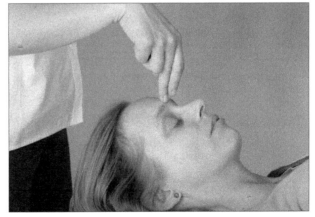

Fig. 3.38 Zhen fa *vibrating* 振法: finger on a point on the forehead.

- A less common yang style method would be elbow Zhen fa, used for strong stimulation of deep points such as Huantiao GB30 and for large muscles.

Historically it is known that some Tui na doctors who were particularly skilled with Zhen fa were able to sustain it for up to 2 hours! I think if you can sustain it for 10 minutes and still feel comfortable, then not only should you feel pleased with yourself but also you will be able to employ Zhen fa to great effect in your practice.

Clinical application and therapeutic effects

Where to apply the technique on the body

Zhen fa can be used anywhere. Finger Zhen fa is commonly applied to any points anywhere on the head or body and to joints. Palm Zhen fa is used on the abdomen, ribs, chest, lower back and sacrum.

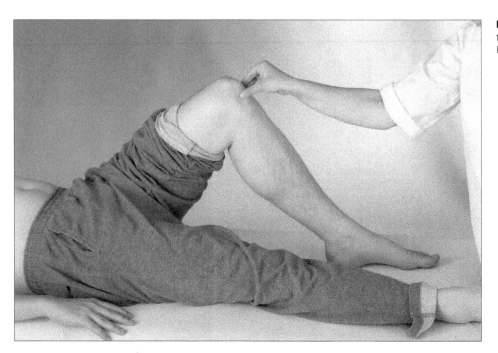

Fig. 3.39 Zhen fa *vibrating* 振法: thumb and middle finger at the knee joint.

Tips for practice

- Relax both body and mind.
- Be aware of your breathing. Do not hold your breath.
- Direct your Qi from the pearl in your Dantian up through your body and then down your arm to your palm or fingers.
- Imagine your dominant arm is a hollow tube and allow Qi to flow through it.
- Use relaxed tension of your muscles.
- Use the weight of your arm and hand.
- Vibrate up and down, not side to side.
- Practice Shaolin Qigong
- Smile, be patient – eventually the vibration will be strong and even.

Therapeutic effects

The penetrating high-frequency vibration produced by Zhen fa has a deep, moving and warming effect on a patient's Qi making it therapeutically flexible. Zhen fa applied to points on the head and face will calm the mind, stimulate the brain and improve the memory and the eyesight.

Used on the abdomen it can warm the Middle and Lower Jiao, regulate the flow of Qi, disperse Blood stasis, clear food stagnation, promote digestion, regulate the Intestines and warm the Uterus.

It can break up accumulations, adhesions and Blood stasis. It opens the chest and aids breathing. It stimulates the functions of the points.

Common uses

- Use Zhen fa on the head, chest and distal points according to the disharmony as part of treatment for insomnia, headaches, anxiety, vertigo, poor memory, dull thinking, poor concentration and poor vision.
- Use palm Zhen fa on the belly, sacrum and relevant Back Shu points for digestive disorders such as nausea, epigastric and abdominal pain, constipation, IBS, a feeling of Fullness and distension, and for gynecological problems such as period pains, fibroids and ovarian cysts, caused by Cold and/or Qi and Blood stasis.
- Use Zhen fa to break up adhesions caused by traumatic injury or surgery. If you want to apply this stronger method of Zhen fa, you will need to add more pressure. I would suggest that you do not attempt this method until you are very comfortable with Zhen fa using just the natural weight of your arm and hand, otherwise there is a danger of forcing it and attempting to use only muscular force rather than Qi.

Che fa *squeezing tweaking*

Che fa is used mainly to stimulate points and sections of the primary channels. It is quite a harsh technique to receive but is therapeutically very effective for expelling Wind-Cold and Wind-Heat from the Wei Qi level and for moving Blood stasis.

How to practice Che fa

Using the ends of the pads of your thumb and index finger, squeeze and pull up the skin and superficial muscles between your finger and thumb; then immediately and quickly release them. Continue working on a point or along a channel at a moderate speed until the skin becomes red.

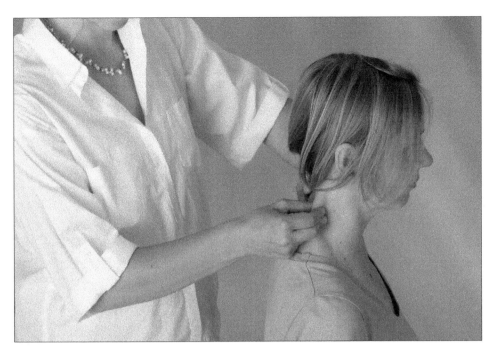

Fig. 3.40 Che fa *squeezing tweaking* 扯法: applied to the neck.

Before you use Che fa on patients, practice on points on your own forearm and hand so you know what it feels like. For added stimulation, add a quick twisting movement as you release the skin. (Fig. 3.40)

Tips for practice

- Squeeze the point evenly between your thumb and index finger.
- After lifting up the skin, immediately release it.
- Do not grip the skin too tightly.
- Try adding a twisting movement when you release the skin, like clicking your fingers.

Clinical application and therapeutic effects

Where to apply the technique on the body

Che fa can be applied to any point on the body but it is most commonly applied to points on the hands and feet, the face, head, neck, chest and along the channels.

Therapeutic effects

It stimulates the actions of the points, expels the pathogenic factors of Wind-Cold and Wind-Heat, aids menstruation and digestion, and disperses stasis.

Common uses

- Use Che fa for external invasions of Wind-Cold and Wind-Heat such as the common cold, flu and hayfever. Choose points that expel these pathogens. For example, if a patient has a Wind-Heat invasion, as part of your treatment you could use Che fa on Quchi LI11 until the point becomes red, then continue to work down along the channel to Hegu LI4 which you can then also stimulate until it is red.

- Che fa is a good technique for getting into the occipital points Fengfu Du16, Tianzhu BL10 and Fengchi GB20 as part of treatment for stiff neck and headaches. Use it on the belly and on related distal points for digestive problems, nausea, motion sickness and blocked menstruation. It is also useful for superficial forms of Bi syndrome.

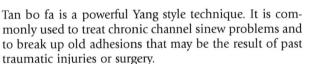

Tan bo fa *plucking* 彈撥法

Tan bo fa is a powerful Yang style technique. It is commonly used to treat chronic channel sinew problems and to break up old adhesions that may be the result of past traumatic injuries or surgery.

Tan bo fa is applied at the analgesic level of treatment after plenty of adaptive work has been done to warm and relax the patient and the superficial tissue layers. It does produce an intense sensation and some patients will find it initially painful to receive.

There are several ways of applying Tan bo fa. In all cases you are plucking over channel sinews, over areas of adhesion, restriction and contracted tendons and muscles.

How to practice Tan bo fa

Always pluck lightly to start with and gradually increase the pressure and intensity of the plucking.

Basic single-thumb plucking

One of the most common methods is to pluck over the area to be treated with the radial side of the pad of the thumb of your dominant hand. Apply pressure to get in and under the adhered muscle or tendon and then pluck across it like plucking a guitar string. Allow the rest of your fingers to naturally relax onto your patient's body. (Fig. 3.41)

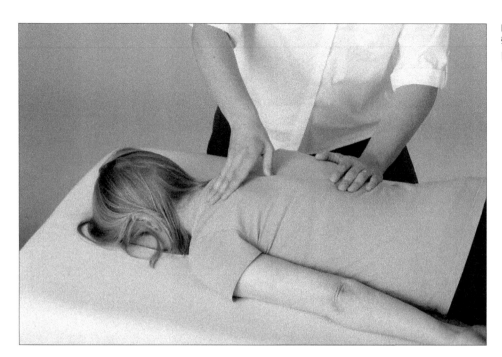

Fig. 3.41 Tan bo fa *plucking* 彈撥法: basic single-thumb plucking.

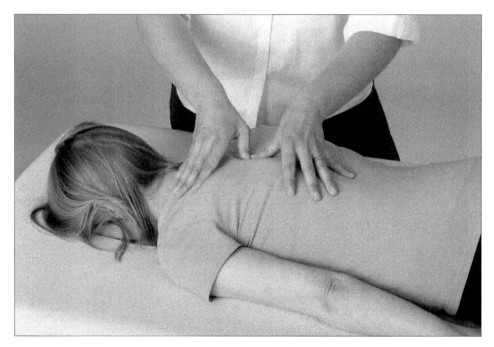

Fig. 3.42 Tan bo fa *plucking* 彈撥法: basic supported-thumb plucking.

Basic supported-thumb plucking

Apply pressure with your dominant thumb trying to get under the contracted or adhered channel sinew. Put your other thumb on top to reinforce the pressure and to apply the force of the plucking. The fingers of both hands should be in contact with the patient's body; this provides support for you and feels reassuring and secure from the patient's point of view. (Fig. 3.42)

Variation of supported-thumb plucking

This method is very useful for working with deep adhesions and if you are applying plucking for relatively long periods of time or on several areas, as it is easier on your thumb.

Bend the distal joint of your dominant thumb to 90 degrees and push in and under the tendon as before with the tip of your thumb; the palm and fingers remain in

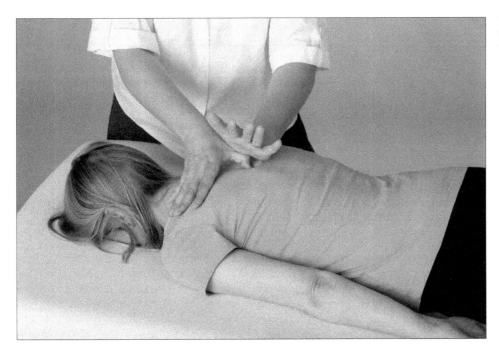

Fig. 3.43 Tan bo fa *plucking*
彈撥法: variation of supported-thumb plucking.

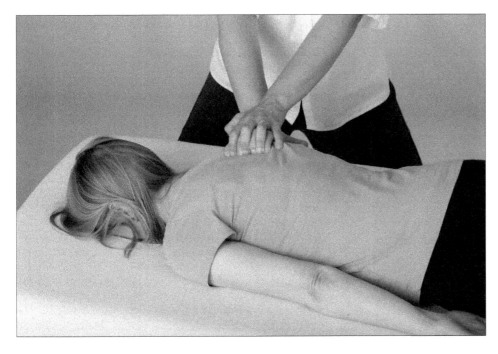

Fig. 3.44 Tan bo fa *plucking*
彈撥法: with the fingers of both hands.

contact with the patient. Use the center of the heel of the palm of your non-dominant hand to apply further pressure onto the bent distal joint. The pressure and momentum for this variation of plucking comes from the non-dominant hand. (Fig. 3.43)

Plucking with the fingers of both hands

Put the palm of your dominant hand onto the patient's body and put the other palm directly on top of it. Bend the distal joints of the four fingers, search out the sinew to be worked on and pluck it towards you. You can also pluck using all eight fingers by putting the fingers of the hand on top in between the fingers of the bottom hand. (Fig 3.44)

Clinical application and therapeutic effects

Where to apply the technique on the body

Tan bo fa can be applied to any channel sinew, and any tendon or muscle that is restricted, contracted, excessively taut or adhered. It is commonly applied to sites of old trauma and the adhesions that have subsequently formed.

Tips for practice

- Remember, Tan bo fa often produces an intense sensation that some would describe as pain, so start gently and gradually increase the intensity of the plucking.
- Work with your patient's breath.
- Even though the technique is quite harsh, keep your Qi and your hands soft.
- Try to get in underneath the sinew then pluck over it like a guitar string.
- Use dispersing techniques frequently when using a lot of Tan bo fa to clear and release stagnant and pathogenic Qi.
- Tan bo fa lends itself well to blending with other basic techniques such as Zhen fa and Rou fa and to passive movements such as Yao fa *rotation*. Experiment and play with this on your fellow students or colleagues.

Example: Try plucking with one thumb over the Large Intestine channel sinew in the forearm, plucking over the sinew and then kneading in an arc until you are back where you started. Repeat this several times in one area, gradually moving along the channel from elbow to wrist. Also, try adding some Yao fa *rotation* to the wrist joint using your non-dominant hand.

Therapeutic effects

Tan bo fa breaks up adhesions and scar tissue. It is a highly effective technique for transforming the shape and structure of the body. It does this by releasing and clearing the channel sinews of deeply held stagnation and stasis, emotional and postural holding patterns.

Common uses

- Use Tan bo fa for any situation where the structure of the body is being compromised by adhesion and contracture of the channel sinews. It is highly effective as part of the treatment for scoliosis in which case it is applied to the Bladder channel sinew and the Huatuojiaji points.
- Use it for the treatment of old traumatic injuries such as sports injuries that have damaged tendons and ligaments.
- Used in the groin over the Liver and Spleen channel sinews, Tan bo fa is very useful for the treatment of hip problems. In this case use the finger plucking method because you can pluck away from the groin rather than towards it and the palm is safely in contact with the patient's thigh. This way both you and your patient feel more secure and it minimizes the embarrassment often felt when working in this rather intimate area.
- Whenever there is any type of adhesion or scar tissue I would strongly consider Tan bo fa as part of treatment.

Cuo fa *rub rolling*

Cuo fa is generally applied at the end of a treatment to relax the patient and to stimulate and regulate the flow of Qi and Blood and disperse stagnation. It can be applied with the whole palm and fingers of both hands in full contact with the area to be treated or with the major or minor thenar muscles or the heels of the palms, depending on which part of the body you are treating. For example, if you are working along the ribcage, you will need to use the whole of your hands; for the shoulder, the emphasis is on the heels of your hands and major thenar muscles.

Cuo fa is most frequently used on the ribcage to regulate Liver Qi and on the shoulder and upper limb for Wind-Cold-Damp Bi syndrome and aches, pains and injuries of the muscles and tendons. Rub rolling the palm is very useful for local problems of the hands and fingers such as 'trigger finger' and carpal tunnel syndrome.

How to practice Cuo fa

Cuo fa requires the even coordination and strength of both hands. You will have to experiment to see which part of your hands fit best in different areas of the body and on patients of different sizes. Keeping a firm and constant contact with your patient by applying opposing pressure between your hands, rub and roll the area to be treated rapidly and vigorously between your hands, moving gradually and slowly down from top to bottom.

Example – working on the ribcage

With your patient sitting either on the edge of your treatment couch or on a stool, stand behind them in a low and grounded posture. Put your hands either side of their ribcage, just below the armpits. Using the whole palm and fingers of both hands, apply opposing pressure and begin to rub and roll the ribcage rapidly between your hands (think of rolling a large ball). Slowly and smoothly work your way down to the bottom ribs. Cuo fa is quite strenuous to perform on the ribcage so you will be pleased to know that you only need to apply it three times. (Fig. 3.45)

If you are working on the shoulder joint, apply Cuo fa starting from the top of the joint and gradually work your way down the whole arm.

Example – working on the upper limb

Have your patient seated while you sit, kneel or adopt a half squat standing posture to the side of the limb you want to work on. When working on the shoulder, you can either have the patient's arm relaxed at their side or you can support their arm over the top of your shoulder. I adopt the second method with patients who are much bigger than me or who have heavy, bulky muscles. This method lends itself well to coordinating a simple passive movement of the shoulder which is achieved by straightening and bending your knees.

Put one hand on either side of the shoulder with your fingers pointing upwards. Hold the joint loosely between

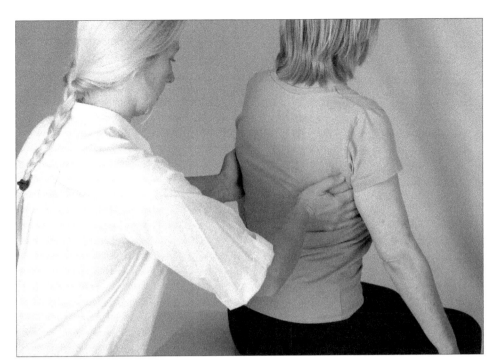

Fig. 3.45 Cuo fa *rub rolling* 搓法: on the ribs.

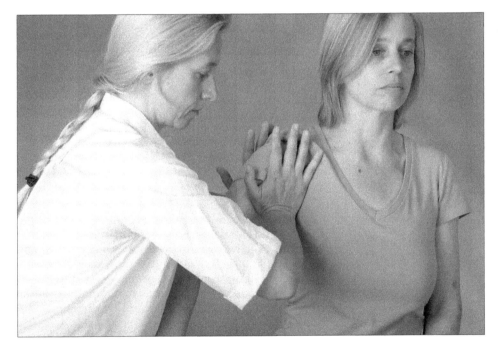

Fig. 3.46 Cuo fa *rub rolling* 搓法: on the shoulder.

the heels of your hands and major thenar muscles. If you have your patient's arm down by their side, lift the joint slightly using the heels of your palms. Now begin to rub and roll the shoulder between your hands quite rapidly. Maintaining a constant pressure and even rhythm, start to move smoothly and slowly down your patient's arm all the way to the hand. If you have their arm supported on your shoulder, when you get to the elbow you will then need to bring their arm down by their side to work from the elbow to the hand. Repeat three times in total, keeping the frequency and pressure even. (Fig. 3.46)

Cuo fa of the palm

Raise your patient's hand and bend their elbow with the back of their hand facing you. Hold the thumb and index finger with one hand and the ring and little finger with your other hand. Rub roll the hand briskly. This method can also be used on the feet. (Fig. 3.47)

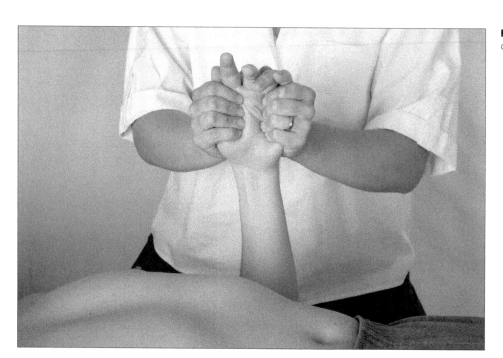

Tips for practice

- Keep a stable grounded posture.
- Rub roll rapidly and move down along the area slowly and gradually.
- The movement should not be too large – keep it neat and controlled.
- Keep a constant, even, opposing pressure between your hands. Do not skim over the surface of the skin.
- Rub roll firmly. Imagine rolling a ball between your hands.

Clinical application and therapeutic effects

Where to apply the technique on the body

You can apply Cuo fa to the ribcage, shoulders, arms, hands, legs and feet.

Therapeutic effects

Cuo fa relaxes tendons and muscles, regulates Qi and Blood flow, disperses stagnation, dredges the channels and collaterals, harmonizes the Middle Jiao, disperses stagnant Liver Qi, aids respiration, moves Blood, eases pain and relieves spasm of tendons and muscles.

Common uses

- Use Cuo fa on the ribcage at the end of your treatments for asthma, a feeling of Fullness and distension in the chest, breathing problems and hypochondriac pain from Liver–Spleen disharmony.
- Use palm Cuo fa for trigger thumb or finger, writer's cramp, numbness of the fingers and hands, Raynaud's syndrome and carpal tunnel syndrome.
- Use Cuo fa on the upper limb for Bi syndrome, frozen shoulder, carpal tunnel syndrome and RSI.

- Use it generally for aches, pains and injuries of the muscle and tendons of the limbs and extremities.

Dou fa *shaking*   抖法

Dou fa *shaking* technique can be applied to the arms and legs. In practice it is often used with Cuo fa *rub rolling*, alternating between the two techniques at the end of a treatment to relax the muscles and joints.

How to practice Dou fa

Example of arm Dou fa

Your patient may be lying down supine or seated. Hold their arm just above the wrist with both hands. Do not grip too tightly. Lift their arm up to just below their own shoulder height and slightly out to the side. Keep your back straight and elbows bent. If your patient is seated, ask them to keep their body weight back and to stay upright. Create a little traction, stretching their arm by dropping your body weight back. Once you have some traction, begin to shake the arm up and down using small controlled movements. The shaking should begin at a moderate speed and build up gradually until it is a very rapid vibration. The shaking should create a wave that transmits all the way up to the shoulder. Shake at least 20 times. (Fig. 3.48)

Example – working on the leg

With your patient lying supine on the treatment couch, stand at the foot of the couch, take hold of your patient's leg just above the ankle with both hands and lift the leg up a little off the couch. Keep your elbows bent and shoulders relaxed; drop your body weight back so that you can stretch the leg, creating a little traction. Now begin to shake the leg up and down with small controlled

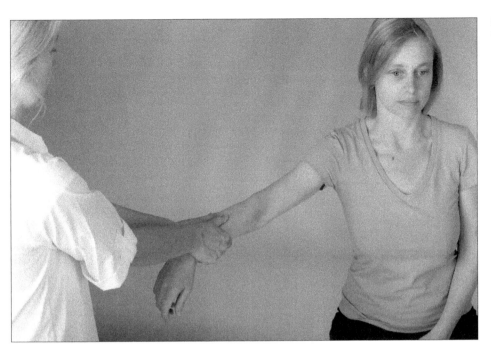

Fig. 3.48 Dou fa *shaking* 抖法: the arm.

movements. Start slowly and build up speed. Try to transmit the wave of vibration up to the hip. Shake at least 10 times. (Fig. 3.49)

Tips for practice

- Use your body weight to achieve traction.
- Keep the shaking small and controlled.
- Start slowly and build up speed until it creates a fast vibration traveling up to the shoulder or hip.
- Try alternating Dou fa with Cuo fa *rub rolling*.

Clinical application and therapeutic effects

Where to apply the technique on the body

Apply Dou fa to the arms and legs.

Therapeutic effects

Dou fa regulates the flow of Qi and Blood throughout the limbs, relaxes the muscles and joints and removes obstructions from the channels.

Common uses

- Use Dou fa towards the end of treatment for muscular/sinew problems of the limbs, aches and pains due to injuries and RSI.
- Use it for Bi syndrome, frozen shoulder, tennis elbow and generally for joint problems of the hip, knee, shoulder and elbow.

Gua fa *scratching/scraping* 刮法

Gua fa is very similar to ancillary therapy gua sha (see p. 113). Instead of using a gua sha board you use your hands. It is applied with the tips of your fingers and thumbs in the gesture of an eagle's claw directly to the skin using talc, water or an external herbal formula such as white or red flower oil. It will produce redness on the skin surface but not the characteristic 'rash' produced by gua sha.

It works on the Wei Qi level and has two main functions. First, it releases the Exterior, expelling external invasions of Wind-Cold, Wind-Heat and Damp. I nearly always include Gua fa as part of treatment for common colds and flu. Second, it strengthens and warms Wei Qi and invigorates Yang.

How to practice Gua fa

Have your patient lying prone. Apply a suitable massage medium such as talc to your patient's back. Adopt the gesture of an eagle's claw with your hands and put the tips of your fingers and thumb of your dominant hand onto your patient's upper back. Line your middle finger up to Dazhui Du14 and arrange your other fingers and thumb either side of the spine in contact with the Bladder channel. Bring your mental focus and Qi to your fingers and scratch down the Governing Vessel forcefully and quickly from top to bottom. When you have finished one downward stroke with your dominant hand, immediately start scratching down with your other hand. Repeat like this using one hand after another. Gua fa needs to be both fast and forceful to be effective. Stop when you feel your patient's skin is scorching hot. After working on the Governing Vessel, repeat the scratching either side of the spine down the Bladder channel, first to the left side and then to the right. Repeat until scorching hot as before. (Fig. 3.50)

Clinical application and therapeutic effects

Where to apply the technique on the body

Gua fa is most commonly applied to the back and waist; it can also be used on the channels of the arms and legs.

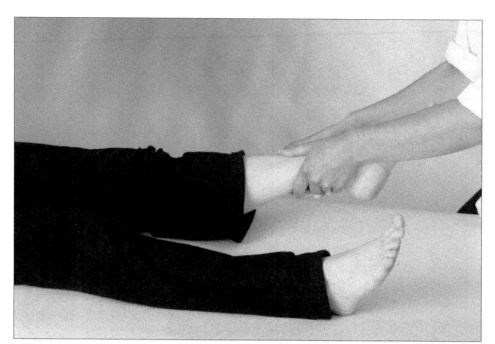

Fig. 3.49 Dou fa *shaking* 抖法: the leg.

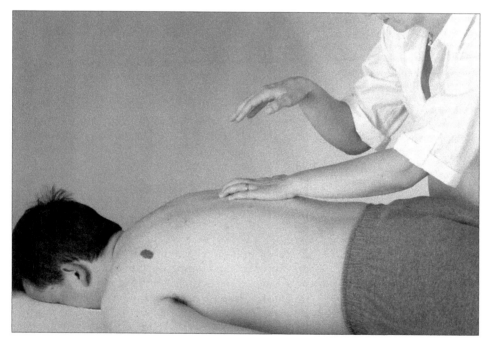

Fig. 3.50 Gua fa *scratching/ scraping* 刮法: on the back.

Tips for practice

- Think of a dog scratching at the earth.
- Keep it fast and forceful.
- Use the pads of your fingers. Do not scratch with your nails.
- Apply to the skin surface using a massage medium.
- Keep going until the skin is scorching hot.

Therapeutic effects

Gua fa releases the Exterior and expels Wind-Cold, Wind-Heat and Damp. It strengthens Wei Qi, invigorates and warms Yang, particularly Spleen- and Kidney-Yang. It warms the Middle Jiao, expels Cold and helps to eliminate Damp. It relaxes the muscles, dredges the channels and harmonizes Qi and Blood.

Common uses

- Use Gua fa for all external pathogenic invasions such as the common cold and flu. Use it to strengthen the immune system of patients who frequently and easily get coughs and colds and so on.
- Use it for digestive disharmonies due to Spleen-Qi and Spleen-Yang Xu, Cold and Damp.

- Use it for muscular aches and pains and backache especially if there is Kidney-Yang Xu or Damp and Cold in the channels. When using Gua fa to strengthen Kidney-Yang, apply it from the waist to the sacrum using a warming medium such as red flower oil.
- Gua fa can also be used to move obstructions and can help with constipation, difficulty urinating and problems due to Blood stasis such as fibroids.

Ca fa *scrubbing*

Ca fa is applied directly to bare skin using some form of external herbal massage medium. Done correctly, this scrubbing technique produces incredible heat; when applied with the minor thenar eminence, it will make the skin scorching hot.

Dong qing gao ointment and woodlock oil are both popular massage media to use with Ca fa, especially in the treatment of muscular skeletal problems. Pure talcum powder can also be used to help resolve Damp and toasted sesame oil to strengthen the Spleen and muscles.

How to practice Ca fa

Ca fa is a dynamic technique requiring strong shoulder muscles; it takes a bit of practice and regular Shaolin Qigong to get it just right!

Depending on what and where you are treating you can apply Ca fa using:

1. The whole palm
2. The minor thenar muscle and ulnar edge of the little finger
3. The major thenar muscle

Ca fa is performed from a standing position. Keep in a low posture with your knees bent and your feet either 1.5 × shoulder width apart or adopt a half lunge position with your front leg bent and back leg straight.

Example using whole palm

First apply a little dong qing gao or other massage medium to the patient's back. Put the whole of your palm and fingers down onto the right-hand side of the Bladder meridian of the back, keeping your fingers together. Now, using the strength of your shoulder muscles, drive your hand forwards along the channel until your arm is fully lengthened, then pull your arm and hand straight back. This is one cycle. Keep your hand in contact with the skin surface at all times. The movement should be as large as you can make it with no downward pressure. (Fig. 3.51)

Example using minor thenar muscle and ulnar side of little finger

As before, apply some dong qing gao or other massage medium to the patient's sacrum. Using your minor thenar muscle and the ulnar side of your little finger, scrub forwards and backwards in straight lines over the patient's sacrum using the strength of your shoulder muscles; do this up to 10 times or until the skin feels scorching hot. Keep your fingers held together. (Fig. 3.52)

Example using the major thenar muscle

This version is great for the limbs. Apply a massage medium to the Stomach channel in the thigh. Put your major thenar muscle onto Biguan ST31 and scrub back and forth between here and Liangqui ST34.

The strength and force are in the forwards and backwards movement. Start gently and slowly and gradually

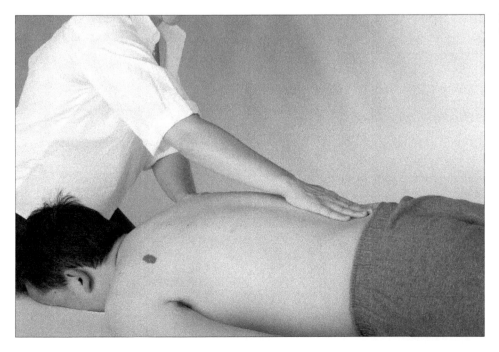

Fig. 3.51 Ca fa *scrubbing* 擦法: whole palm on the back.

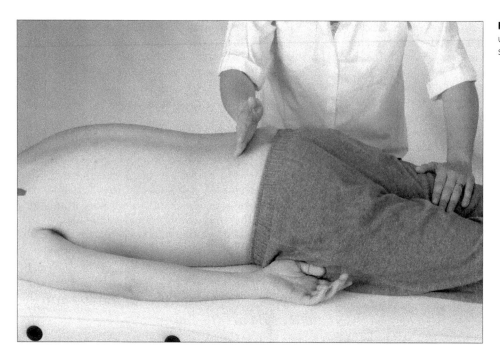

Fig. 3.52 Ca fa *scrubbing* 擦法: ulnar edge of hand on the sacrum.

increase your speed. There should be no downward pressure, only the natural weight of your arm, as this will prevent the production of the desired heat. The rate of Ca fa is about 100 cycles per minute, but you only need to do 10 cycles to any one area. Any more than this and the skin becomes too hot and you could create blistering or scalding.

Tips for practice

- Think of polishing a huge wooden table.
- Keep your hand in contact with the skin at all times.
- Start gently and slowly and increase your speed.
- Make the backwards and forwards movement big and straight.
- Do not press downwards.
- Let the drive come from your shoulder.
- Apply about 10 times until the area is hot.

Clinical application and therapeutic effects

Where to apply the technique on the body

Ca fa can be applied to the back, chest, abdomen, arms and legs. Use the whole palm for large areas, such as the back, chest and abdomen. Use the major thenar muscle for the legs and arms and the minor thenar muscle and ulnar side of the little finger for the sacrum and the Huatuojiaji points.

Therapeutic effects

Ca fa warms the channels, removes obstructions from the channels and activates the circulation of Qi and Blood. It eases pain, expels Wind and Cold, reduces swelling, relieves oppressive and stuffy feelings in the chest and will strengthen the Zangfu.

In practice I have also found Ca fa useful to draw retained pathogenic Heat to the surface in cases such as recurring colds and flu. In these cases I would apply Ca fa to the Governing Vessel from Dazhui Du14 down to Mingmen Du4 using the minor thenar muscle and a cooling medium such as white flower balm or talc.

Common uses

Common uses for Ca fa are:

- Lower backache and sciatica
- Bi syndrome
- Muscular skeletal aches and pains
- Trauma and injuries
- Deficiency of Qi and Blood
- Deficient conditions of the Zangfu
- Common cold
- Retained and trapped pathogens
- Qi stagnation
- Cough
- Cold patterns and Yang Xu

Ca fa is generally used at the end of a treatment or just before the use of passive movements such as Ba shen fa *stretching*, Yao fa *rotation* and Ban fa *twisting*.

CHAPTER **4**

Compound techniques

The basic techniques are like an artist's pallet of colors. Some lend themselves particularly well to blending. Compound techniques are essentially either two basic techniques blended together, such as Na fa *grasping* with Rou fa *kneading* to form kneading–grasping, or a basic technique blended with an action like holding or pinching, for example Na fa blended with pinching gives us pinching–grasping.

There are undoubtedly many possible ways to create compound techniques and I encourage you to explore the various possibilities in practice groups with fellow students and colleagues. However, there are 13 compound techniques that have developed over Tui na's long history that are most commonly used and are especially useful in clinical practice. It is these that I will focus on in this chapter. Na fa and Rou fa, the most flexible basic techniques, are used in all but two of the 13 compound techniques.

As students of Tui na, learning and mastering these techniques will help you develop the sophistication and flow of your techniques and confidence and sensitivity in your hands. As Tui na practitioners, the compound techniques provide us with greater subtlety in our art and flexibility in practice.

In this chapter I will give a description of how to apply each technique, where it can be applied on the body, its therapeutic effects and indications for its use in treatment.

Compound techniques using Na fa

There are seven compound techniques that use Na fa as the root technique. They are:

1. Holding–grasping
2. Pinching–grasping
3. Grabbing–grasping
4. Nipping–grasping
5. Plucking–grasping
6. Lifting–grasping
7. Pulling–grasping

1. Holding–grasping

Holding–grasping makes use of the whole hand to hold, squeeze and grasp the muscles and channel sinews.

Attach the whole of your palm and fingers to the area to be worked on, hold and squeeze the underlying muscles and then add the grasp, which lifts the underlying tissues away from the bone. Hold and grasp the muscles firmly and suddenly, keeping the palm of your hand in full contact, and then release the muscles so that your hand is no longer touching. Do not be tempted to rush this technique; it needs to be applied at a steady pace allowing time to pause briefly in between.

Holding–grasping can be applied repeatedly in one particular area such as the deltoid muscle, or along the course of the channel's sinews. You can use one or both hands depending on the area to be treated and the size of your patient. (Fig. 4.1)

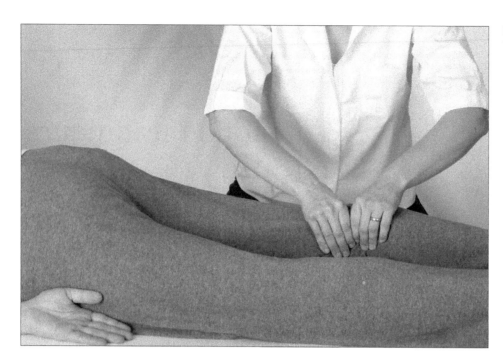

Fig. 4.1 Holding–grasping on the backs of the legs.

Clinical application and therapeutic effects

Where to apply the technique on the body

Holding–grasping is most commonly applied to the muscles and channel sinews in the shoulders, arms, hips and legs. It can also be applied to the neck, back and around the waist.

Therapeutic effects

Holding–grasping is a comfortable technique to receive. I often use it at the end of the adaptive stage of treatment before applying some of the more intense and stimulating compound blends of Na fa.

Holding–grasping warms the channels and dredges the channels and collaterals. It can be used to release the Exterior, expel Wind and disperse Cold. It will relax the muscles, alleviate pain, invigorate Qi and Blood and eliminate stasis.

Common uses

Apply holding–grasping to the back of the neck to stimulate the Bladder and/or Gallbladder channels then apply several times along the course of the relevant channels in the arms and legs as part of treatment for common colds, flu, headaches and dizziness.

Use for muscular stiffness and spasm, Wind-Damp-Cold Bi syndrome, Wei syndrome and difficulty walking. Use for any disharmony caused by Cold, Qi stagnation and Blood stasis.

2. Pinching–grasping

Pinching–grasping is applied with the thumb on one side of a muscle or channel sinew and all four fingers on the other side. It can be applied using either one hand or both hands working side by side.

Pinch the muscle between the pads of your thumb and fingers, add the grasping to lift the muscles and then immediately let go, completely releasing the muscle, and then repeat. By adding pinching to grasping it produces quite intense stimulation.

This technique should feel deep and penetrating but not harsh; there must be softness within it. Keep a relaxed soft focus on what you are trying to achieve; keep your breath centered and even and use only the pads of your fingers, not the tips or nails.

Pinching–grasping can be applied with consistent repetition in one fixed place or along the course of a channel. It should be applied until the patient feels a sensation of soreness, numbness or distension. (Fig. 4.2)

Clinical application and therapeutic effects

Where to apply the technique on the body

Pinching–grasping can be applied to most muscles and channel sinews. It is most commonly applied to both the Yin and Yang channels of the arms and legs.

Therapeutic effects

These are wide and varied as it depends on which channels are being stimulated.

- When applied to the Yin channels of the arms it will help to clear the Lungs, stop a cough, resolve Phlegm, aid respiration and calm the Shen.
- Applied to the Stomach, Spleen and Liver channels it can help to regulate and encourage digestion.
- When applied to the leg channels, it will move Qi and Blood in the abdomen.
- Generally, pinching–grasping will invigorate the flow of Qi and Blood, relax the muscles and open the channels.

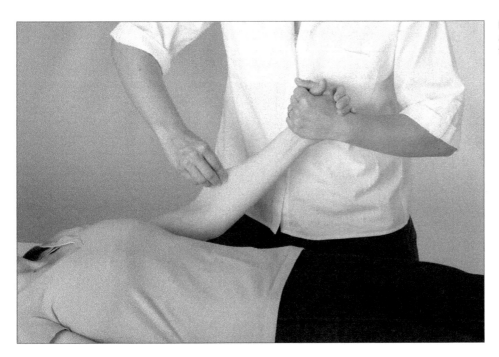

Fig. 4.2 Pinching–grasping along the Lung channel in the forearm.

Try moving from holding–grasping to pinching–grasping for stronger stimulation in the analgesic stage of treatment.

I find this a very flexible and effective compound technique, useful for a wide range of conditions. While working along a channel you can pause at important points relevant to the treatment along the way and focus the technique there for a minute or so before moving on.

Common uses

- Include pinching–grasping in your treatment of mental/emotional problems such as anxiety, depression, panic attacks and palpitations.
- You can use it for respiratory conditions such as asthma, acute and chronic cough and difficulty breathing due to retention of Phlegm.
- Use it for feelings of oppression in the chest and ribs from Phlegm or Qi stagnation.
- Apply to the leg channels for digestive problems such as hiccup, belching and flatulence, abdominal pain and distension caused by Shi conditions and for dysmenorrhea from Qi stagnation and Blood stasis.

3. Grabbing–grasping

Grabbing–grasping is applied with the tips of the fingers and thumb of one or both hands. The palm is empty, making no contact with the body.

Create an eagle's claw posture with your hand. Bring your Qi to the tips of your fingers and thumb and grab the area to be worked on like an eagle grabbing its prey; add grasping by lifting the underlying muscles and then quickly release them. Repeat rhythmically in one place or along the course of the channels.

When applying to the head, have your patient seated and stand to one side. Support your patient's forehead with your non-dominant hand. Apply grabbing–grasping with your dominant hand by spreading your clawed fingers so that the middle finger is in line with the Governing Vessel; your index and ring fingers are either side in line with the Bladder channel and your thumb and little finger with the Gallbladder channel. Grab and grasp from the anterior hairline working gradually backwards.

When applying to the abdomen, follow the patient's breath, either by grabbing and grasping during the in breath and releasing with the out breath, or by applying several times during the out breath.

Grabbing–grasping is quite an intense technique: keep relaxed, brisk and rhythmic; use your Qi and do not let it become harsh. (Fig. 4.3)

Clinical application and therapeutic effects

Where to apply the technique on the body

Grabbing–grasping can be applied to the head, neck and nape, the back, abdomen, arms and legs.

Therapeutic effects

Grabbing–grasping is a dispersing technique. It has a powerful effect on Wei Qi and can be used to release the Exterior, expel Wind, disperse Cold and drain Damp. It warms the channels, relaxes muscles and channel sinews and invigorates and moves Qi and Blood. It can be used to promote urination and to stop pain.

Common uses

Grabbing–grasping can be used for any type of channel sinew problem, muscular stiffness, spasm or pain from backache to stiff neck. Specifically:

- It is definitely worth considering in cases where you have Wind obstructing the channels creating stiff

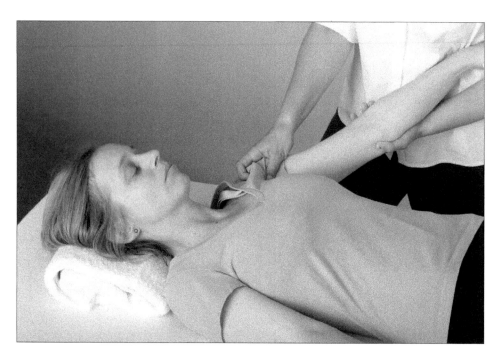

Fig. 4.3 Grabbing–grasping on the shoulder.

contracted sinews in the arms and legs. For example, you may see extreme cases of this in cerebral palsy and multiple sclerosis (MS) when the legs or arms cannot be straightened.

- It can also be used as part of treatment for headaches and migraine, common cold and flu.
- It is a useful technique to apply to the belly for abdominal pain from stasis of Blood and retention of Cold or Cold and Damp.
- It can be used as part of treatment for diarrhea caused by Cold and Damp patterns with Weak Spleen.
- It can also help in cases where flow of urine is impeded or blocked by accumulations and stagnation.

4. Nipping–grasping

Using the tips of your fingers and thumb, nip a point or several points around a joint by pressing into it with your fingers and thumb, grasping and then releasing. Nip and grasp energetically and repetitively until the Qi is strongly stimulated and the patient feels a sore, numb, aching sensation.

Clinical application and therapeutic effects

Where to apply the technique on the body

Nipping–grasping is mainly applied to joints and points and any depressions and fossas. It is very useful for stimulating points at the occiput like Tianzhu BL10 and Fenchi GB20. I use it between vertebrae to stimulate the Governing Vessel.

It is commonly applied to the neck and nape, the shoulders, elbows, wrists, knees and ankles. (Fig. 4.4)

Therapeutic effects

Nipping–grasping is used to expel Wind, disperse Cold, move Blood and disperse Blood stasis; it dredges the channels of obstructing pathogens and stagnated Qi. It relieves pain, relaxes the channel sinews and opens and lubricates the joints by bringing Qi and Blood to them.

Common uses

Nipping and grasping is very useful in the treatment of arthritis, Bi syndrome from Wind-Damp-Cold, traumatic injuries and any restricted joint movement such as frozen shoulder. I have found it useful in the treatment of carpal tunnel syndrome and repetitive strain injury (RSI).

5. Plucking–grasping

Plucking–grasping is applied with the pads of the thumbs and fingers. The two most common ways of applying this compound technique are:

1. Grasp a tendon firmly between the pads of your thumb on one side and your fingers on the other, lift the tendon up away from the underlying bone and pluck it evenly between your fingers and thumb; imagine plucking a double bass string. You can apply this method with one hand or both hands working side by side. You can work in one area such as the extensor tendon at the lateral epicondyle of the humerus, plucking and grasping the Large Intestine channel sinew, or you can work gradually along the channel sinew. (Fig. 4.5)
2. Grasp the tendon or channel sinew between the pads of your thumb and fingers and pluck over the tendon with your thumb, like plucking a guitar string.

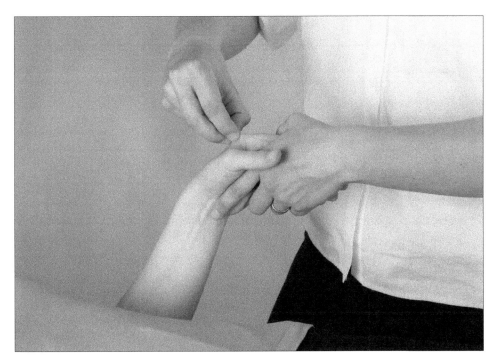

Fig. 4.4 Nipping–grasping Hegu LI4.

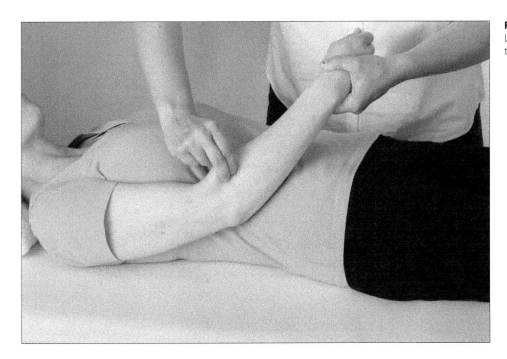

Fig. 4.5 Plucking–grasping the Large Intestine channel sinew in the forearm.

With either of these methods, do not work too quickly. Give yourself time to search out areas of adhesion and feel the quality of the tissue under your fingers.

Clinical application and therapeutic effects

Where to apply the technique on the body

Plucking–grasping can be applied to any channel sinew where tendons are prominent. It is most commonly applied to the sinews in the neck and nape, the shoulders, the back, arms and legs.

Therapeutic actions

Plucking–grasping is an intense technique and like other forms of Tan bo fa it is not the most pleasant technique to receive. Its therapeutic effects come about through intense repetitive stimulation, which aims to break up adhesion of the tendons and fibrous muscle tissue. It can be very effective at doing this.

It dredges the channels, and relaxes and rectifies tendons and sinews. It expels Wind, drains Damp and disperses Cold. It moves Qi and Blood, breaks up stasis and helps to alleviate pain.

Common uses

Plucking and grasping can be used in the treatment of most channel sinew problems; it is particularly useful in cases where there is a history of traumatic injury. The Blood stasis caused by these injuries is often untreated and the patient often presents with adhesion, muscular spasm, numbness and restricted movement. It is used frequently to treat stiff neck, backache and Wind-Damp-Cold Bi syndrome.

6. Lifting–grasping

There are two methods of applying lifting–grasping:

1. Using both hands, grasp and lift up the muscles using the pads of your fingers and thumbs and then, keeping the muscles lifted, roll them forwards and then backwards several times until they become warm. This method can be applied to the abdomen and ribs or along the spine working either from the sacrum to the nape or vice versa depending on the treatment principle. (Fig. 4.6)
2. Grasp and lift the muscles of the abdomen between the pads of your thumbs and fingers, then while the muscles are lifted, twist them back and forth quickly several times and then release. Repeat this until you or your patient feels a sensation of warmth in the area. This method is applied to the muscles of the abdomen and ribs. (Fig. 4.7)

Do not apply lifting–grasping harshly, keep softness in your hands and mind and take care not to grasp the internal organs when working on the abdomen.

Clinical application and therapeutic effects

Where to apply the technique on the body

Lifting–grasping is most commonly applied to the muscles of the abdomen and ribs and along the spine.

Therapeutic effects

Lifting–grasping will help to regulate the digestion, harmonize the Middle Jiao, move stagnant Liver Qi and soothe the Liver. It warms and disperses Cold, strengthens the Spleen and Stomach and regulates the intestines. When applied to the spine from the sacrum to Dazhui Du14 it strengthens Spleen- and Kidney-Yang. It can alleviate pain, relax muscle spasms and dredge and clear obstructions from the channels.

Common uses

Lifting–grasping is a very useful compound technique to include in the treatment of digestive disorders. It is particularly useful in cases of stagnation of Liver Qi and Middle Jiao disharmony with Wood overacting on Earth causing symptoms such as hypochondriac pain and distension, irritability, depression, IBS, hiccups and belching. It can be used for acute abdominal pain caused by Cold and Qi stagnation, for diarrhea from Spleen- and/or Kidney-Yang Xu and for acute backache.

7. Pulling–grasping

Pulling–grasping is applied to joints and the sinews around them. One hand pulls to create joint traction and to stretch the associated tendons and muscles, while the other hand applies either basic Na fa or an appropriate

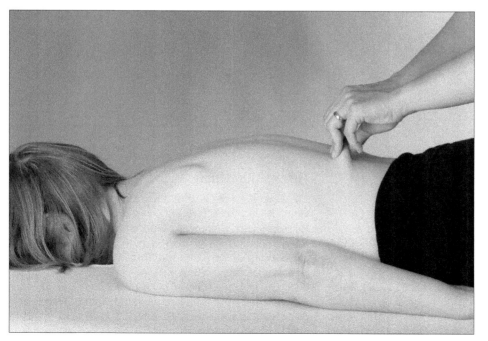

Fig. 4.6 Lifing–grasping along the spine.

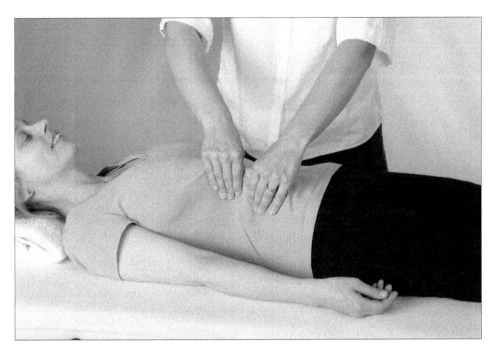

Fig. 4.7 Lifting–grasping on the abdomen.

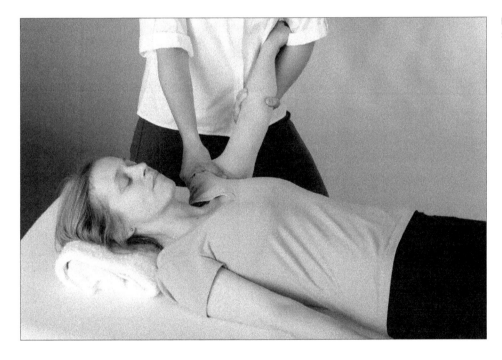

Fig. 4.8 Pulling–grasping the shoulder joint.

compound blend such as pinching–grasping, grabbing–grasping, holding–grasping, nipping–grasping or kneading–grasping to the affected channel sinews around the joint. (Fig. 4.8)

Clinical application and therapeutic effects

Where to apply the technique on the body

Pulling–grasping is most commonly applied to the neck, shoulders, elbows, wrists, fingers, knees, ankles and toes.

If you are working with an assistant or a team of practitioners, you can work together to apply pulling–grasping to the back, waist and hips. To do this, one practitioner holds either one or both legs just above the ankle, and leaning backwards, uses their body weight to pull and create traction. While the traction is applied the other practitioner works on the local areas by grasping the sinews of the back, waist or hips.

Therapeutic effects

Historically, the setting of fractured or broken bones was an important specialist area of Tui na and there are still Tui na doctors in some traditional Chinese medicine (TCM) hospitals in China who specialize in bone setting. Pulling–grasping is one of the techniques that are employed for this purpose.

In a 21st century Western Tui na practice we do not treat broken bones and fractures. Pulling–grasping is used to relax and rectify the channel sinews, to relieve muscle spasm, open and lubricate the joints and increase the range of their movement. It is used to bring Qi and Blood to traumatized joints and channel sinews, to dissipate Blood stasis, reduce swelling and alleviate pain.

Common uses

Pulling–grasping can be used as part of treatment for traumatic injuries to the joints and channel sinews with restricted joint movement. It is commonly used in the treatment of wry neck, cervical spondylosis, frozen shoulder, tennis elbow, pain around the scapula, RSI, sprained wrists and ankles, stiff back, lumbar strain and prolapsed lumbar discs.

Compound techniques using Rou fa

There are four compound techniques that use Rou fa kneading as the root technique. They are:

1. Kneading–grasping
2. Kneading–pinching
3. Kneading–nipping
4. Kneading–vibrating

1. Kneading–grasping

Kneading–grasping is applied with the palm, fingers and thumb of one or both hands. Keep the center of your palm in contact with the area to be treated and knead and grasp the muscles in a circular motion. The kneading and grasping is driven by the elbow and wrist, which need to remain fluid and flexible. The grasping is applied with the bellies of your fingers and thumbs. The knack is to keep the technique fluid, moving around and along the channel sinews being treated.

Clinical application and therapeutic effects

Where to apply the technique on the body

Kneading–grasping is a very flexible compound technique; it is most commonly applied to the neck and back, the arms and legs, shoulders and hips, and abdomen. (Fig. 4.9)

Therapeutic effects

Kneading–grasping is a comfortable technique to receive and its flexibility makes it very useful in practice. It can be used as an adaptive technique in the early stages of treatment to relax the sinews and the patient generally. It is equally useful as a dissipative technique that you can keep coming back to during treatment. It can be used to expel Wind, disperse Cold, and resolve Damp and to dredge the channels. It moves Qi and Blood, disperses Blood stasis and alleviates pain.

Common uses

Kneading–grasping can be used as part of treatment for external invasions of Wind, Wind-Cold and Wind-Damp-Cold.

For common cold, flu, headache and stiff neck apply kneading and grasping to the neck and nape, shoulders and generally along the Tai yang and Shao yang channel sinews.

Kneading–grasping is very effective in the treatment of Wind-Damp-Cold Bi syndrome causing symptoms like backache, soreness and aching of the muscles and joints, numbness and restricted joint movement. It is also used in the treatment of traumatic injuries to help to stop swelling and move Blood stasis.

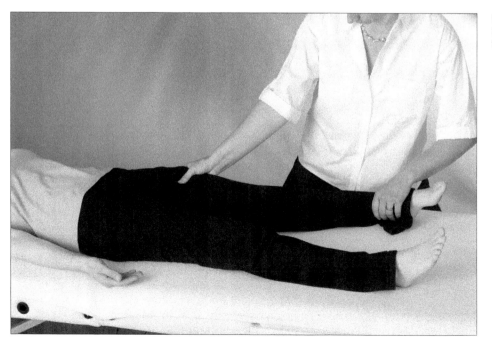

Fig. 4.9 Kneading–grasping the Stomach channel sinew on the thigh.

2. Kneading–pinching

Knead and pinch using the pads of your thumb and fingers. The palm of your hand is not involved. You can use all of your fingers or any combination of fingers depending on the size of the area being treated. For example, you only need to use your thumb and index finger if you are working on a patient's eyebrows. Using one or both hands, knead and pinch the muscles or tendons to be worked on in a circular motion.

Blending in the pinching makes this a penetrating technique, which is more intense in sensation than the previous kneading–grasping, so keep relaxed and flexible in your fingers, hands and arms, and work with softness.

Clinical application and therapeutic effects

Where to apply the technique on the body

Kneading–pinching can be applied continuously in one place for several minutes or you can work gradually along the course of a channel. It can be applied to most areas of the body and commonly to the channel sinews of the neck, shoulders, arms, legs, back, chest and face. (Fig. 4.10)

Therapeutic effects

Kneading–pinching is very effective for dispersing and clearing Wind-Damp-Cold and dredging and warming the channels. In practice I have found it very helpful in cases where there is a lot of Damp or Phlegm obstructing the channels.

Applied to points on the face and along appropriate channels such as the Pericardium and Liver, it can be used to calm the mind. Kneading–pinching invigorates and regulates the flow of Qi and Blood; it can disperse Blood stasis, reduce swelling and alleviate pain.

Common uses

- Kneading–pinching is an invigorating, dispersing technique.
- Use it for the common cold and stiff neck to expel Wind or Wind-Cold invasions.
- It is very useful in cases where there is dizziness, muzzy head, nausea and vomiting and the patient is tired and listless.
- Use it in any situation where Damp is present and Qi is obstructed, such as numbness and aching in the body. I have found it useful for MS when there is a weak Spleen and lots of Damp obstructing the channels of the legs. In these cases apply on the back along the Bladder channel and to the Stomach, Spleen, Large Intestine and Lung channels and to any local areas such as the face.
- Kneading–pinching can be used for Wind-Damp-Cold Bi syndromes and backache and traumatic injuries.

3. Kneading–nipping

Kneading–nipping is applied with the tips of the thumb and fingers but not the nails, which will injure the skin. You can use any number of fingers along with your thumb. For example, if you are stimulating a point in an area with large muscles, such as the shoulders or thighs, you will need to use all of your fingers, whereas if you are working on points on the hands or feet you will only need to use your index and possibly middle finger.

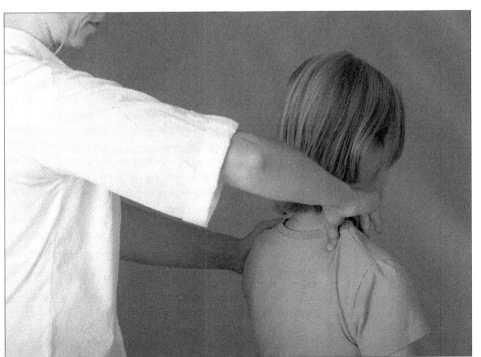

Fig. 4.10 Kneading–pinching the top of the shoulder at Jianjing GB21.

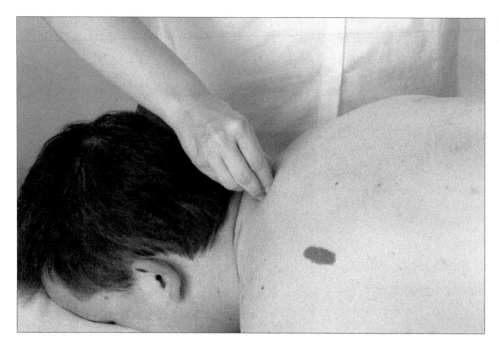

Fig. 4.11 Kneading–nipping Du14.

Press into the point you want to stimulate with the tips of your thumb and fingers. Knead and nip the point in a circular motion; start slowly and gently and gradually increase the intensity and speed. Kneading–nipping is applied continuously until the patient feels a sore, numb sensation at the point and sometimes along the channel. (Fig. 4.11)

Clinical application and therapeutic effects

Where to apply the technique on the body

Kneading–nipping is applied to points and channels.

Therapeutic effects

Kneading–nipping is essentially a point-stimulating compound technique. It is used to stimulate the actions of points, making it therapeutically versatile.

It stimulates at the Wei Qi level and if used on a regular basis can strengthen Wei Qi. Because it is used at points it also penetrates into the primary channels and connects to Ying Qi and can be used to harmonize Yin and Yang.

If applied along the course of a channel it can be used to dredge the channels and collaterals and to promote the flow of Qi and Blood.

Common uses

Depending on the chosen points' prescription, kneading–nipping can be used as part of treatment for any Zangfu disharmony. This is Tui na working in much the same way as acupuncture.

It will help to strengthen Wei Qi if applied regularly to the Governing Vessel from Yaoshu Du2 up to Dazhui Du14 paying particular attention to Mingmen Du4 and Du14, along the Bladder channel from Tianzhu BL10 to Pangguanshu BL28 and along the primary leg channels of the Stomach and Spleen and the arm channels of the Lung and Large Intestine.

It can be used in the treatment of Bi syndrome, Wei syndrome and traumatic injuries.

4. Kneading–vibrating

There are two common methods of applying kneading–vibrating:

1. Using a finger or thumb
2. Using the palm or the major/minor thenar eminence

Applying kneading–vibrating using a finger or thumb

Use either the tip of your middle finger, index and middle finger or the thumb of your dominant hand. Put your finger or thumb onto the point or area to be treated and bring the hollow palm of your non-dominant hand down beside it. Hold the finger or thumb just above the distal joint between the thumb and index finger of your non-dominant hand. Apply some pressure to the point with your finger or thumb and then, staying at that depth, begin to apply Zhen fa *vibrating*; at the same time apply Rou fa *kneading* with your non-dominant hand. (Fig. 4.12)

Applying kneading–vibrating using the palm or the major/minor thenar eminence

You can use either the major or minor thenar eminence, the heel of the palm or the whole palm depending on the area to be treated. Use whichever feels the most comfortable. Knead and vibrate with your dominant hand or, for extra support, put your non-dominant hand on top.

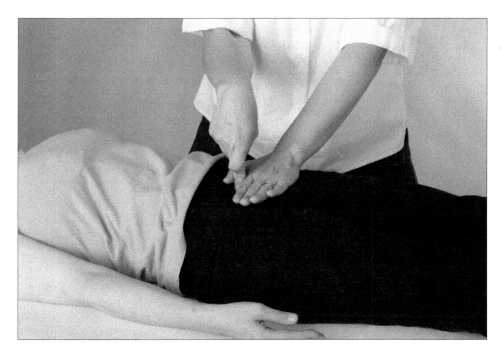

Fig. 4.12 Kneading–vibrating using the middle finger on Guanyuan Ren4.

Clinical application and therapeutic effects

Where to apply the technique on the body

Kneading–vibrating with the fingers or the thumb is mainly used to stimulate points and to work directly on accumulations and masses. It is very useful for working on points on the neck and throat.

Kneading–vibrating using the various parts of the palm is most commonly applied to the back, shoulders, hips, ribs, chest and abdomen.

Therapeutic effects

Kneading–vibrating is a dissipative technique that can penetrate deeply. Therapeutically it is mainly used for breaking up, dispersing and moving both Qi stagnation and Blood stasis. It is used to soften and break up accumulations, masses and adhesions and to warm and dredge the channels.

Common uses

- Kneading–vibrating is great for moving Qi stagnation so you can use it to treat problems like plum stone throat, a feeling of Fullness in the chest, Middle Jiao disharmony, hypochondriac pain and retention of food.
- It is commonly used to treat points on the neck and throat for wry neck, stiffness of the channel sinews, restricted neck movement, voice problems, sore throat and thyroid imbalances.
- Kneading–vibrating can be used to break up old adhesions including scar tissue.
- Use it for backache and traumatic injuries of the limbs and joints as it helps to clear the swelling created by Blood stasis. Try applying it to the tenderest points on the outer Bladder channel around the scapula for whiplash injuries.

- In my experience it is a very useful compound technique to apply in the treatment of gynecological conditions such as fibroids and ovarian cysts. I frequently use it to stimulate coalescent points of the Chong Mai on the abdomen as part of treatment for menstrual disorders such as dysmenorrhea, irregular menstruation and excessive menstrual bleeding.

Other compound techniques

There are two further compound techniques that are commonly used in practice:

1. Pushing–pressing
2. Whisking–sweeping

1. Pushing–pressing

Pushing–pressing is applied with the tips of the middle, index and ring fingers, with most of the emphasis on the middle finger.

Relax, center your breath in your Dantian and ground your energy. Flex the distal joints of your fingers slightly and bring your attention and Qi into your fingers, particularly your middle finger. Work into the fossa to be treated by pushing and pressing up and down, forwards and backwards and from side to side alternately.

Start slowly and gently and gradually increase your speed and pressure. Apply until the patient feels a sensation of warmth and soreness. (Fig. 4.13)

Clinical application and therapeutic effects

Where to apply the technique on the body

Pushing–pressing is applied to the subclavicular fossa, the axilla and the popliteal fossa. When applying it to the

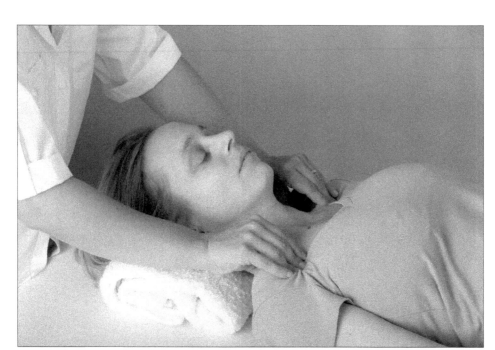

Fig. 4.13 Pushing–pressing applied to the subclavicular fossa.

subclavicular fossa, stand or sit at the head of the patient who is lying prone and work on both sides at the same time.

Therapeutic effects

- Applied to the subclavicular fossa, pushing–pressing has a powerful ability to descend rebellious Qi, particularly rebellious Lung and Stomach Qi.
- Applied to both the subclavicular fossa and the axilla it moves stagnant Qi, dissipating and relieving feelings of Fullness and distension in the chest, hypochondria, epigastrium and abdomen.
- Applied to the popliteal fossa it will increase movement in the knee joint, relax muscular spasms affecting the Bladder channel sinew, alleviate pain and clear febrile heat, and Heat from the Blood.
- Apply to all three areas to regulate and harmonize Qi and Blood.

Common uses

- Pushing–pressing can be applied as part of treatment for cough, asthma, oppressive and restricted feelings in the chest, difficulty breathing and retention of Phlegm.
- It can be used in the treatment of hiccups, belching, nausea, vomiting, epigastric pain and distension of the hypochondrium and abdomen.
- Use it for lower backache, lumbar strain, pain along the course of the Bladder channel sinew and inhibited movement of the knee joint.
- You can also use it as part of treatment for urticaria and eczema due to Heat in the Blood, and for febrile diseases to clear Heat.

2. Whisking–sweeping

Whisking–sweeping is applied with the palm and fingers of one hand or both hands together. The key is to keep very relaxed and loose, particularly in your wrist and elbow joints. Put the palm and fingers of one or both hands onto the area to be treated; keep in full contact but do not apply any pressure. Drive the movement from your arms, keeping your wrist completely relaxed and loose and your fingers soft. Whisk your hands back and forth, outwards then inwards in a brisk, light manner. Think of what you would do to warm someone up when they are cold.

Whisk in one area such as the upper back increasing the speed of your whisking gradually, and then sweep your hands out and away firmly with the intention of clearing what you have dissipated. You can work like this in one area or along a channel, whisking many times repetitively and then sweeping away firmly. (Fig. 4.14)

Clinical application and therapeutic effects

Where to apply the technique on the body

This compound technique is most commonly applied to the upper back and shoulders and to the lumbar area around the waist. Several of my colleagues and I use whisking–sweeping all around the ribcage and down the Yang channels of the arms and legs.

Therapeutic effects

Whisking–sweeping is a dissipative technique that is often applied at the end of a treatment for general dissipation and during treatments after the application of a technique that produces deep intense stimulation.

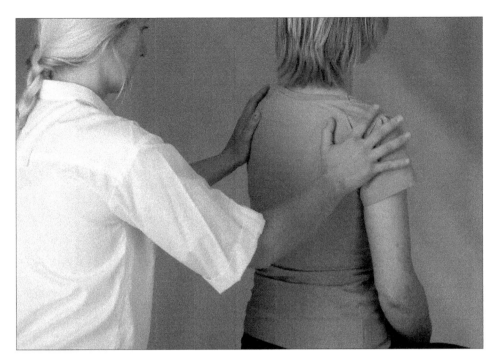

Fig. 4.14 Whisking–sweeping the upper back.

It is used to expel Wind and disperse Cold, to clear Damp and to resolve Phlegm. It is used to clear the Lungs and open the chest to warm the channels and to alleviate pain.

Common uses

- Whisking–sweeping is gently invigorating and is very effective for patients who are both Qi Xu and Damp, and feeling tired and weak. I frequently use it at the end of treatment to dissipate any released pathogens and stagnation and to invigorate the patient.

- It can be used in the treatment of respiratory problems such as coughs, stuffy chest, wheezing and asthma, especially when there is retention of Phlegm.
- I use whisking–sweeping on the ribcage in the treatment of Liver Spleen disharmony to move the Qi stagnation, warm the Spleen-Qi and to drain Damp.
- It is also commonly applied in the treatment of back pain, and Wind-Damp-Cold Bi syndrome.

CHAPTER **5**

Coordinated techniques

Coordinated techniques are essentially two different techniques, basic or compound, applied at the same time to stimulate two areas of the body simultaneously. Think of rubbing your tummy and patting your head. About 70% of the Tui na treatments I give involve coordinating two techniques in some way and I have several colleagues who do the same. It is a very effective and practical way of working.

Tui na can be time-consuming; techniques need to be applied for long enough to allow their particular vibratory frequencies to penetrate and their therapeutic qualities to emerge. Working with two techniques at the same time means that you can work locally and distally simultaneously, for example working on a local area such as the lower back with one hand and on a distal area such as a point on the Bladder channel in the calf with the other hand.

In a modern Western practice, if you are working on your own and your patient can only come say once a fortnight, working in this way means that you can cover more and maximize the use of the treatment time.

In theory, as long as you can perform the techniques fluently, you can coordinate any two techniques together: a basic technique with a compound technique, two basic techniques or two compound techniques. As you gain more confidence and experience of working with Tui na you will discover and develop your own particular favorite and effective combinations. When you feel confident and fluid with the basic and compound techniques, I would encourage you to explore and experiment with various combinations as they arise. There are many possibilities and variations.

In this chapter I will describe 11 coordinated techniques. I have included some classic combinations that are frequently employed in Tui na departments in China, some variations of these classics, and a few combinations that my colleagues and I use frequently and have found to be very useful in practice. These techniques are:

1. Gun fa and Rou fa
2. Gun fa and An fa or Ya fa
3. Gun fa and Pai fa
4. Gun fa and Yi zhi chan tui fa
5. Gun fa and Tui fa
6. Forearm Rou fa and pinching–grasping
7. Elbow Rou fa and Ji dian fa
8. Loose first Pai fa and pinching–grasping
9. An fa and Mo fa
10. Whisking–sweeping and Pai fa/Ji fa
11. Pai fa/Ji fa and Ji dian fa

1. Gun fa and Rou fa

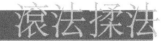

Clinical application and therapeutic effects

Where to apply the combination on the body

This is a very flexible combination and can be applied to most areas of the body. It is commonly applied in the following ways:

1. Applying one technique to the lower back, sacrum and hips and the other down the back of the legs along the Bladder/Gallbladder channels.
2. Applying one technique on the abdomen and the other down the leg along the Stomach channel.
3. Applying one technique to the hip with one hand and the other technique to the shoulder with your other hand.
4. Applying Rou fa with one hand to a point with the thumb or middle finger and Gun fa with the other hand along a channel or section of a channel.

How to apply the combination

Below are examples of how to apply the first three of the above four methods of application. The fourth I think speaks for itself. Work with these methods until you feel comfortable applying Rou fa and Gun fa at the same time, then try experimenting and you will discover other ways. Keep the ones that work for you.

Applying to the lower back, sacrum and hips and down the back of the leg

Stand to one side of your patient and apply Rou fa to the lower back, sacrum and hips using either your forearm, palm, the heel of your palm, major or minor thenar eminence. Use whatever feels most comfortable. The forearm is very useful for working over large muscles such as the psoas and gluteus and for working over the Governing Vessel and Back Shu points.

Apply Gun fa with your other hand working gradually along the Bladder channel from the area of Chengfu BL36 down to Kunlun BL60 and then back up again. You can also apply the techniques the other way around, using Gun fa at the lower back, sacrum and hips and Rou fa down the legs. (Fig. 5.1)

Applying to the abdomen and along the Stomach meridian in the leg

Adduct your patient's leg slightly so that their toes are pointing inwards; this exposes the Stomach channel. One hand performs Rou fa on the abdomen, which can be applied in several different ways. You can use your palm or forearm over major abdominal points or you could use your thumb or middle finger to stimulate abdominal points.

While one hand applies Rou fa to the abdomen, the other applies Gun fa along the Stomach meridian working from Biguan ST31 to Jiexi ST41.

It is also possible to apply Gun fa to the abdomen along the Stomach channel, for instance, and to apply Rou fa to distal points in the leg. (Fig. 5.2)

Applying to the hip and shoulder

Standing to one side of your patient who is lying prone, apply Rou fa with your palm, heel of your palm, forearm or elbow to the area of Tianzong SI11 and Gun fa to the area of Huantiao GB30. Then swap and apply the techniques the other way around.

Therapeutic effects

Gun fa and Rou fa can be used to expel Wind-Damp-Cold, strengthen the Stomach and Spleen, harmonize the Middle Jiao, warm and strengthen Kidney-Yang, eliminate Damp, promote urination and bowel movement, soften, release and nourish the channel sinews, move Blood and resolve stasis, warm and dredge the channels and alleviate pain.

Common uses

Bi syndrome, backache and aching muscles and joints, traumatic and sports injuries, Wei syndrome, weakness of the limbs, Kidney-Yang Xu, poor digestion, Liver–Spleen

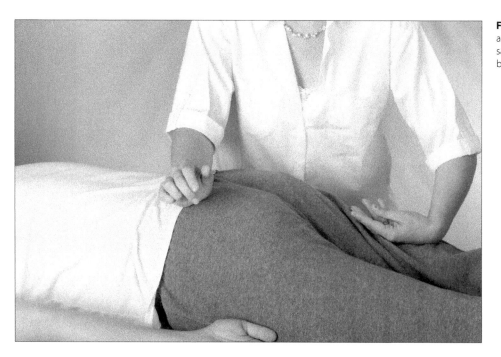

Fig. 5.1 Gun fa and Rou fa applied to the lower back, sacrum and hips and down the back of the leg.

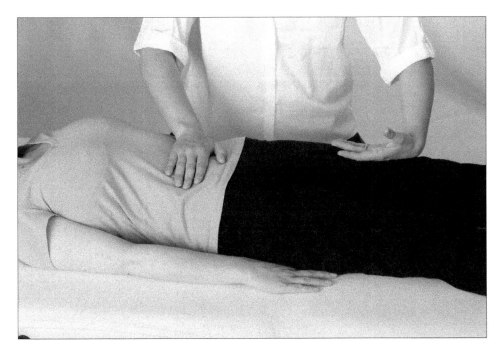

disharmony leading to irritable bowel syndrome (IBS), acute and chronic epigastric and abdominal pain, Spleen and Stomach Qi Deficiency and menstrual problems such as dysmenorrhea and irregular menstruation.

2. Gun fa and An fa or Ya fa 滾法按法壓法

Clinical application and therapeutic effects

Where to apply the combination on the body

This combination is used to stimulate points using An fa with the thumb or Ya fa with the elbow and to work along a section of a channel using Gun fa with the other hand. Here are some common methods of application:

- Applying An fa with your thumb to a point on one side of the back while the other hand performs Gun fa on the opposite side
- Applying Ya fa with your elbow to points in the lower back, hips and thighs while the other hand applies Gun fa along a leg Yang channel (Fig. 5.3)
- Applying Gun fa to the back, hips and sacrum while the other hand stimulates distal points using An fa
- Applying An fa to points in the forearm while the other hand applies Gun fa to the shoulder

How to apply the combination

I will describe how to apply the first two methods. When you feel at ease with them, explore coordinating Gun fa and An fa or Ya fa in a variety of different ways. Be creative!

Applying An fa to a point on one side of the back while the other hand performs Gun fa on the opposite side

With your patient lying prone, stand at their head. Using the thumb of one hand, apply An fa to points at the top of the right shoulder and upper back; the Huatuojiaji and Back Shu points are a good place to start. Apply Gun fa with your other hand to the top of the left shoulder and the left side of the nape and upper back, stimulating the Tai Yang channel sinews. Repeat on the other side.

Applying Ya fa with your elbow to points in the lower back, hips and thighs while the other hand applies Gun fa along a leg Yang channel

Choose a Yang channel point to stimulate in the lower back, hip or upper thigh. Apply Ya fa to the point with your elbow and at the same time apply Gun fa back and forth along the related Yang leg channel.

Therapeutic effects

An fa and Ya fa stimulate the individual actions and spirits of the points so this combination has great versatility.

This combination is often used to: open the chest and aid respiration when applied to the upper back, nape and shoulders; to move and dissipate stagnation of Qi and Blood stasis; to soften, release and relax the tendons and muscles; to facilitate joints; to warm and dredge the channels.

Common uses

This combination can be used for: channel sinew problems such as muscular pain, stiffness, aching and weakness, restricted joint movement, Bi syndrome, Wei syndrome, traumatic injuries, menstrual problems and

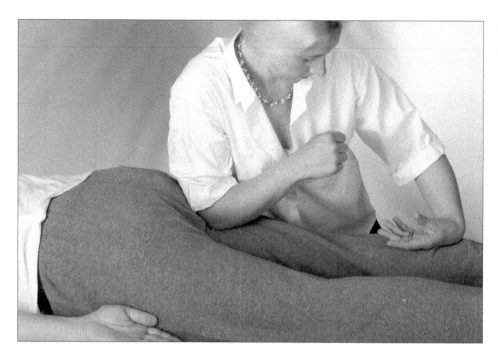

Fig. 5.3 Ya fa BL36 and Gun fa on the calf along the Bladder channel.

gynecological conditions caused by Qi and Blood stasis and Cold. It is also used for respiratory problems such as asthma and cough.

3. Gun fa and Pai fa 滚法拍法

Clinical application and therapeutic effects

Where to apply the combination on the body

The most common methods of application are:

- Gun fa down one side of the Bladder channel of the back and Pai fa down the other side
- Pai fa over the lower back and hips and Gun fa along the course of the Bladder or Gallbladder channels of the legs; or the other way round
- Pai fa on the abdomen and Gun fa down the Stomach channel of the leg

How to apply the combination

A description of how to apply the first and third methods follows.

Gun fa down one side of the Bladder channel of the back and Pai fa down the other side

Standing at the head of your patient, apply Gun fa to one side of the Bladder channel working gradually from the nape down to about the level of the waist, if you can reach. With your other hand apply cupped palm Pai fa to the Bladder channel on the other side. Repeat the other way round. (Fig. 5.4)

Pai fa on the abdomen and Gun fa down the Stomach channel of the leg

Stand to one side of your patient and apply Pai fa to their abdomen working either in clockwise circles or in lines

along the channels; you can also apply Pai fa to the rib-cage area.

At the same time apply Gun fa along the Stomach channel of the leg. Repeat, working from the other side of the body. You can also use Gun fa on the abdomen, working in lines along the channels, and apply Pai fa down the legs and or arms.

Therapeutic effects

Gun fa with Pai fa is a very effective coordinated technique to use for clearing and dredging the channels of obstructing Damp and Phlegm and generally for dissipating any stagnation and stasis of Qi and Blood. It opens the chest, expels and clears Wind-Damp-Cold, helps to descend rebellious Qi, relaxes the channel sinews and eases spasm and alleviates pain.

Common uses

This combination can be used for: respiratory problems such as wheezing, asthma, difficulty breathing, cough with retention of Phlegm and an oppressive feeling in the chest, Bi syndrome, Wei syndrome, muscular aching and stiffness, any Middle or Lower Jiao problems involving Damp and/or rebellious Qi such as nausea and vomiting, IBS, ulcerative colitis and ovarian cysts.

4. Gun fa and Yi zhi chan tui fa 滚法一指禅推法

Clinical application and therapeutic effects

Where to apply the combination on the body

This combination is very flexible and can be applied to the back, hips, neck and nape, shoulders, arms, legs, chest and abdomen.

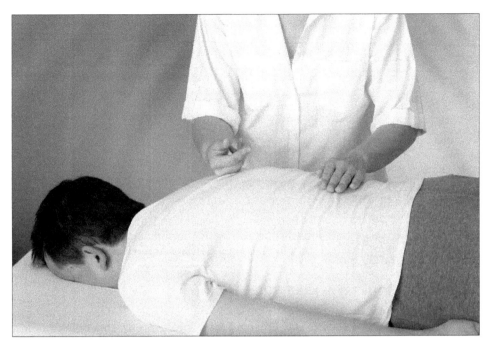

Fig. 5.4 Gun fa and Pai fa on the back.

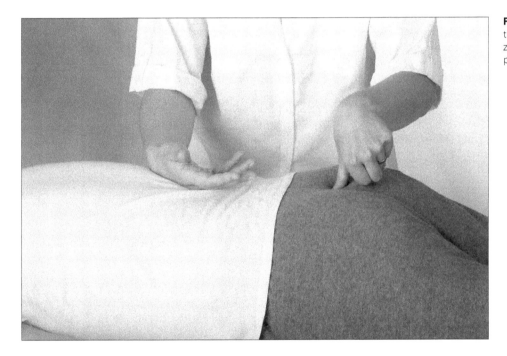

Fig. 5.5 Gun fa and Yi zhi chan tui fa: Gun fa to the waist, and Yi zhi chan tui fa to a sacral foramen point.

How to apply the combination

Once you have mastered Yi zhi chan tui fa and Gun fa you can have some fun practicing using them at the same time. This combination is so powerful that you could give a whole treatment using this combination alone.

Choose a point to be stimulated and apply Yi zhi chan tui fa to the point with one hand. At the same time apply Gun fa with your other hand to a local area or along a channel. Try applying this combination in as many ways as you can think of.

Example for practice

Apply Gun fa to the waist, concentrating on stimulating the inner and outer Kidney Back Shu points; at the same time apply Yi zhi chan tui fa to one of the sacral foramen points. This would be useful not only for lower back problems, but also for menstrual disorders and gynecological problems that are related to Cold, Damp, Qi stagnation and Blood stasis. (Fig. 5.5)

Therapeutic effects

The individual natures of the points are activated with Yi zhi chan tui fa while Gun fa warms and activates, moves and dredges, depending on your intention and the manner in which you apply it.

Common uses

This combination is very wide ranging and could be applied as part of a treatment for most disharmonies including: Bi and Wei syndrome, channel sinew problems, Zangfu disharmonies leading to a variety of problems from digestive disorders to menstrual and fertility problems.

5. Gun fa and Tui fa 滚法推法

Clinical application and therapeutic effects

Where to apply the combination on the body

This combination is most commonly applied in the following ways:

- Applying Gun fa to the lower back, sacrum and hips while the other hand applies Tui fa to the Bladder or Gallbladder channels of the legs (Fig. 5.6)
- Applying Gun fa to the Bladder channel of the leg and Tui fa with the knuckles to the sole of the foot
- Applying Gun fa to the Stomach channel in the thigh and Tui fa down the Stomach channel in the lower leg using the thumb

How to apply the technique

I think the above methods are fairly self-explanatory so I will just explain the second method and let you work the others out for yourself.

Applying Gun fa to the Bladder channel of the leg and Tui fa with the knuckles to the sole of the foot

Standing to the right side of your patient, stand on your right leg and put your left leg, knee bent, onto the bench so that you can put your patient's lower leg onto your thigh. Apply Gun fa to the Bladder channel in the calf with your right hand and apply Tui fa with the knuckles of your left hand to the sole of the foot, stimulating Yongquan KD1.

Therapeutic effects

This combination warms and dredges the channels of obstructing pathogenic factors, activates and moves Qi and Blood, softens, releases and relaxes the muscles.

Common uses

This combination can be used for: lower backache, sciatica, channel sinew problems, Bi and Wei syndrome and Lower Jiao problems caused by Damp and Cold, and Qi and Blood stagnation.

6. Forearm Rou fa and pinching–grasping 揉法

Clinical application and therapeutic effects

Where to apply the combination on the body

Forearm Rou fa is generally used on the back or the abdomen, while the compound technique pinching–grasping is applied to the Yin and Yang channels of the arms and legs.

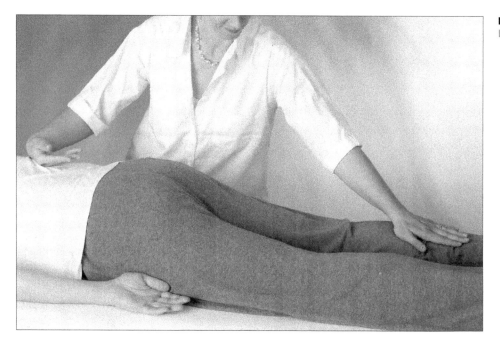

Fig. 5.6 Gun fa and Tui fa on the lower back and leg.

How to apply the combination

You can sit or stand to perform this combination; try both ways and then go with whatever feels more comfortable. When you start practicing, try getting the forearm Rou fa working first. When that is flowing and you feel completely relaxed with it, start to add the pinching and grasping with your other hand. Experiment with pinching and grasping along different Yin and Yang channels. Try the following example.

Forearm Rou fa on the abdomen and pinching–grasping the Stomach and Spleen channels of the leg

Sit or stand to the left side of your patient and apply forearm Rou fa to their abdomen using your right forearm. Focus around the area of Zhongwan Ren12 until it is nice and warm and then work over the navel to stimulate Tianshu ST25. With your left hand, pinch and grasp along the Stomach channel of their left leg working from Biguan ST31 down to Jiexi ST41; repeat several times and then pinch and grasp up the Spleen channel from around Shangqiu SP5 up to Chongmen SP12. Repeat this on the other side, applying Rou fa with your left forearm and pinching–grasping with your right hand.

Therapeutic effects

This combination is very effective for clearing Phlegm from the Lungs, descending Lung-Qi and moving Qi stagnation from the chest. It will disperse Liver-Qi, harmonize the Stomach and Intestines and help to strengthen the Spleen. It can regulate menstruation, activate Blood and move stasis. It strengthens Kidney-Qi, alleviates pain, relaxes muscular tension and spasm and can help to relieve convulsions.

Common uses

This combination can be used for:

- Cough and difficulty breathing due to retention of Phlegm, uncomfortable and oppressive feelings in the chest, chest pain and palpitations
- Epigastric and abdominal pain and bloating caused by retention of food, Liver–Spleen disharmony and Qi and Blood stagnation
- Wei syndrome, backache, Kidney-Qi Xu, soreness and aching of the muscles, irregular menstruation, menorrhagia and amenorrhea

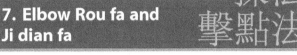

7. Elbow Rou fa and Ji dian fa

Clinical application and therapeutic effects

Where to apply the combination on the body

This combination is generally applied to points in the back, buttocks and legs.

How to apply the combination

The elbow Rou fa stimulates a point in a local area where there are deep points and large muscles, while the other hand applies Ji dian fa to a distal or other relevant point. Try the following example.

Applying to the buttock and lower leg

With your patient lying prone, apply elbow Rou fa to Zhibian BL54 and Ji dian fa with your other hand to Weizhong BL40. Experiment with this combination, trying a variety of different points in the back, buttocks and lower legs. (Fig. 5.7)

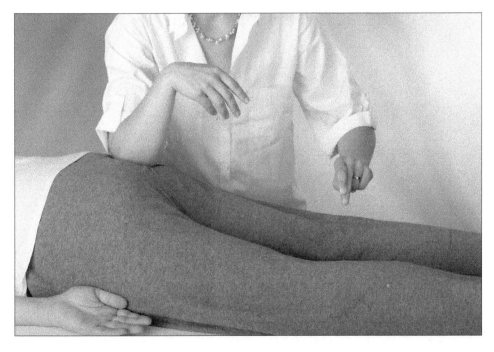

Fig. 5.7 Elbow Rou fa and Ji dian fa: Rou fa on Zhibian BL54 and Ji dian fa on Weizhong BL40.

Therapeutic effects

This combination will relax and release the channel sinews, move Qi and Blood and resolve stasis, open and dredge the channels, disperse Liver-Qi, expel Wind, eliminate Cold and alleviate pain.

Common uses

Elbow Rou fa and Ji dian fa is a very effective combination for rheumatism and rheumatoid arthritis, Bi syndrome of the back and hip, Wei syndrome, pain of the back and legs due to trauma, restricted joint movement of the hip and knee, sciatica and chronic pain and weakness and restricted movement due to old bone traumas.

8. Loose fist Pai fa and pinching–grasping

Clinical application and therapeutic effects

Where to apply the combination on the body

This combination is most commonly applied to the head and the top of the shoulders and to the Yin and Yang channels of the arms and legs.

How to apply the technique

This coordinated combination is generally performed quite briskly. It can be applied in two ways, either by performing both techniques at the same time or by alternating your hands, applying Pai fa then pinching–grasping.

Two examples of how to apply Pai fa and pinching–grasping follow.

Applying to the head and shoulders

Stand behind your patient who is seated. Apply loose fist Pai fa to the vertex of your patient's head using the ulnar edge of your hand. At the same time, with your other hand, pinch and grasp the top of your patient's trapezius muscle, working to stimulate Jianjing GB21 and the surrounding area. Swap hands and repeat on the other side. Coordinate your hands so that you are performing both techniques at exactly the same time. (Fig. 5.8)

Applying to the Yang channels of the arm and leg

Sit or stand to one side of your patient who is lying down on one side with their arms and legs straight. With one hand, apply loose fist Pai fa using your knuckles along the Yang channels of your patient's leg and pinching–grasping with your other hand working along the Yang channels of their arm. Work with the techniques in an alternating rhythm. Try it with the techniques the other way round and then repeat on the other side.

To treat the Yin channels of the arms and legs you will need to adjust the position of your patient a little. They will still lie on one side but facing upward slightly. If they are lying on their right side, stretch out their right arm with the palm facing upwards. Their legs need to be slightly bent and separated so that the Yin channels of the right leg are exposed. Work along the Yin channels as described above.

Therapeutic effects

This combination can be used to harmonize Yin and Yang, move the Blood, dredge the channels, relax the channel sinews, disperse Cold and alleviate pain.

Common uses

It is most commonly used as part of treatment for headaches and migraine and Wei syndrome.

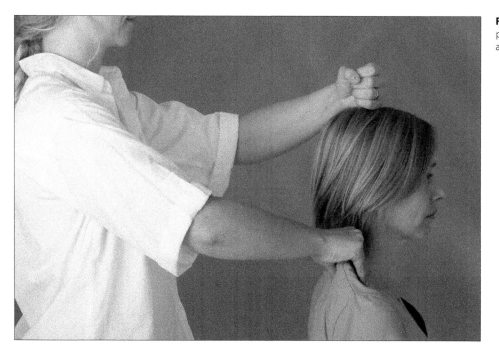

Fig. 5.8 Loose fist Pai fa and pinching–grasping on the head and shoulders.

9. An fa and Mo fa 按法摩法

Clinical application and therapeutic effects

Where to apply the combination on the body

This is a very flexible, coordinated combination that I use frequently in practice. An fa can be applied to any points relevant to the disharmony being treated or along a channel, while Mo fa is applied to the abdomen, ribcage, chest, back, or along the course of the Yin or Yang channels of the arms and legs.

How to apply the combination

I think this is fairly self-explanatory as both of these basic techniques are relatively simple to apply. Try An fa and Mo fa in as many ways as you can think of. To give you somewhere to start, I have listed a few of the methods of application that I find particularly useful and effective:

- An fa using your thumb or middle finger on distal Kidney channel points and Mo fa with the palm of your other hand over Shenshu BL23 and Zhishi BL52. This method is effective for tonifying Kidney Yin and Yang. (Fig. 5.9)
- Mo fa over the Zhongfu LU1 and Yunmen LU2 area and An fa using your thumb along the Lung channel from Chize LU5 to Taiyuan LU9 then resting at LU9 with An fa. This method is effective for tonifying Lung-Qi, descending Lung-Qi and clearing Phlegm.
- Mo fa on the abdomen and An fa on distal Stomach and Spleen channel points to harmonize the Stomach and Intestines and tonify Stomach- and Spleen-Qi.

Therapeutic effects

These are very wide and varied according to the points chosen and how the An fa is applied to stimulate them. Generally though this combination is very effective for tonifying, strengthening and supporting what is weak and insufficient, for warming what is Cold, and for calming the Shen.

Common uses

The clinical uses of the An fa and Mo fa combination are again very varied and include:

- Digestive problems due to Xu patterns, Cold and Qi stagnation, IBS, diarrhea, constipation
- Menstrual disorders from Qi and Blood Xu, Cold and stagnation
- Fertility issues due to Deficiency and Cold
- Respiratory problems such as asthma and chronic cough, tiredness, insomnia, anxiety and depression

10. Whisking–sweeping and Pai fa/Ji fa 拍法擊法

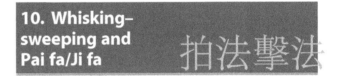

Clinical application and therapeutic effects

Where to apply the combination on the body

This is generally applied to the back and the legs.

How to apply the combination

One hand performs the compound technique whisking–sweeping while the other hand applies Pai fa using either of the loose fist methods and then Ji fa using the ulnar

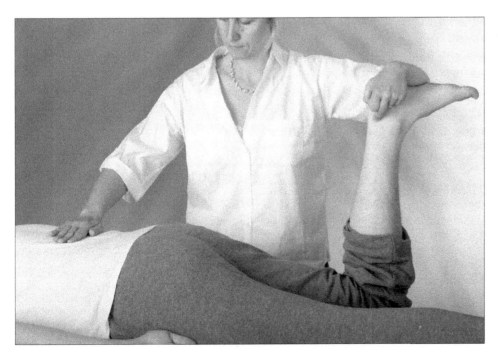

Fig. 5.9 An fa and Mo fa: An fa on KD3 and Mo fa on BL23.

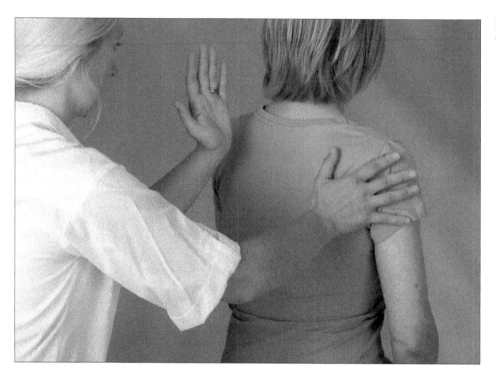

Fig. 5.10 Whisking–sweeping and Pai fa/Ji fa on the back.

edge of the palm. Move between the two striking techniques while the other hand continues to whisk and sweep. Two examples of this combination follow.

Applying whisking–sweeping and Pai fa/Ji fa to the back

With your patient seated, either sit or stand in a low posture behind them. Apply whisking–sweeping to the right side of your patient's upper back and scapula area with your right hand and apply Pai fa and Ji fa to the left side of their back. Work briskly and do not let the striking techniques become too heavy. (Fig. 5.10)

Applying whisking–sweeping and Pai fa/Ji fa to the legs

Starting with your patient lying prone, apply the striking techniques to the back of their upper thigh and whisk and sweep the calf to warm and dredge the Bladder channel. Then ask your patient to lie on their side and apply the striking techniques to the hip and the lateral side of the thigh with one hand and whisking–sweeping to the lateral side of the lower leg with the other hand to warm and clear the Gallbladder channel; repeat.

Finally, ask your patient to lie supine, turn their toes inwards slightly to expose the Stomach channel and apply Pia fa and Ji fa to the upper thigh and whisking and sweeping to the lower leg.

Therapeutic effects

This combination is used to encourage the smooth flow of Qi through the channels and collaterals; it is very effective for clearing feelings of Fullness and distension. It moves Blood, warms and dredges the channels, relaxes the muscles and expels Wind.

Common uses

This is a very useful dispersing combination to use in clinic either towards the end of treatment or when you need to dredge obstructions from the channels during the analgesic stage. Use it for any problems involving Qi stagnation such as feelings of oppression and distension in the chest, hypochondrium and abdomen. Use it for pain, numbness, aching and stiffness in the joints and muscles.

11. Pai fa/Ji fa and Ji dian fa

拍法擊法
擊點法

Clinical application and therapeutic effects

Where to apply the combination on the body

This combination of all of the striking techniques can be used all over the back, sacrum, shoulders, hips, arms and legs.

How to apply the combination on the body

It can be applied either by using two different techniques at the same time, or applying one striking technique after another in any order, such as Pai fa using a cupped palm followed by Ji fa with joined palms and then with hands separate, followed by Ji dian fa using all five fingers. Any of the striking techniques can be used. The most common methods of application follow.

Applying Pai fa/Ji fa and Ji dian fa to the back and shoulders

With your patient either seated or lying prone, apply the striking techniques in any order to their shoulders and

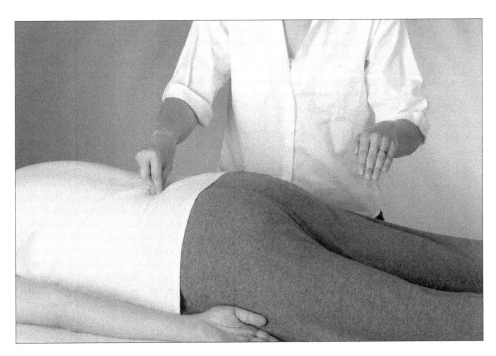

Fig. 5.11 Pai fa/Ji fa and Ji dian fa on the lower back and legs.

back. Work from top to bottom with your hands on either side of the spine. If you are using joined palm Ji fa, strike one side of the back and then the other, crossing over the spine with each strike.

Applying Pai fa/Ji fa and Ji dian fa to the lower back, sacrum and legs

With your patient lying prone, use Pai fa on the lower back and sacrum with a cupped palm. At the same time, your other hand works down the leg along the Bladder channel (Fig. 5.11). Alternate between using three- or five-finger Ji dian fa and loose fist Pia fa with your knuckles. The same method can be applied to the hip and Gallbladder channel with the patient lying on their side.

Therapeutic effects

All striking techniques have the ability to break up and dissipate anything that is stagnant or obstructing. You can use this combination to move Qi and Blood stagnation and to clear Damp and Phlegm.

Common uses

This combination is commonly used for respiratory problems such as cough and asthma, feelings of oppression and distension, stiff joints and muscles, Bi and Wei syndrome, menstrual disorders and digestive problems due to stagnation, stasis and Damp.

CHAPTER 6

Passive movements

A passive movement requires the patient to be passive and relaxed while the practitioner provides movement to the patient's joints, muscles, tendons and ligaments. A passive movement can be anything from a gentle rocking motion to a deep stretch. They are used to take joints and muscles through a range of movements and to the end of their natural range of movement. They provide the body with a reminder of what it can do, nudging it out of the all too often fixed and frozen postural habits that we tend to adopt, through either repetitive work and lifestyle habits or blocked and stagnant emotional energy.

The area of passive movements is extremely wide and varied. I am aware that there are probably as many different schools of thought and approaches to this subject as there are passive movements. Most bodywork systems, whether other traditional Oriental forms such as Thai massage and shiatsu or Western systems like osteopathy, make great use of passive movements, rocking, stretching, rotating and twisting the body back towards a natural state of balance and harmony.

In Tui na practice, passive movements are often integrated into treatment. The type of passive movements used and the way in which they are performed will depend upon the practitioner's style of Tui na and the school of thought that has been passed onto them and that they are influenced by.

Most passive movements fall into the categories of Ba shen fa *stretching* or *traction*, Yao fa *rotating* and Ban fa *pulling* or *twisting*. Both rotation and stretching combine very well with other basic and compound techniques making them very useful and flexible techniques to apply in practice.

Historically, there was a bone-setting school of Tui na. This style of Tui na was the main form of treatment in the bone-setting departments of the Imperial Physicians in the Song (AD960–1279) and Yuan (AD1280–1368) dynasties. The Tui na doctors who worked in this way would use Gao mo, massage with external herbal ointments and passive movements to manipulate and reposition the joints and bones back into place.

Today in the West, patients with broken bones and dislocated joints get treated in the accident and emergency departments of hospitals of Western medicine, so Tui na bone-setting skills are not taught or practiced in the West. In a modern Western Tui na practice, passive movements are generally used to both remove obstructions from the joints and channel sinews and to bring Qi and Blood to them. They are commonly used to treat problems such as stiffness, spasm, restriction and injuries of the joints, muscles and ligaments, Wei syndrome, Wind-Damp-Cold Bi syndrome and deviations of the vertebrae.

There are too many different types and versions of passive movements to include them all in this book. Practitioners have their favorites and many develop their own versions of the classic traditional Chinese medicine (TCM) hospital style passive movements. I have included in this chapter the passive movements that my colleagues and I have found to be practical, safe and useful in today's Tui na practice. At the end of this chapter you will find some general tips for applying passive movements and the contraindications for these techniques.

Ba shen fa *stretching/traction*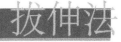

Ba shen fa involves stretching the channel sinews and creating space for joints.

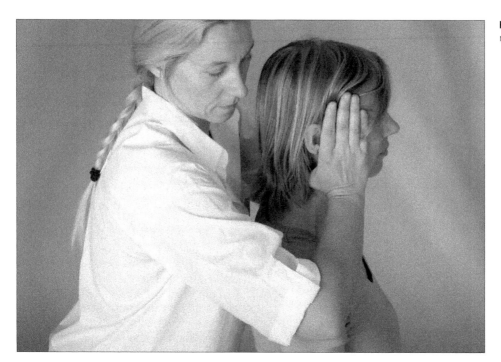

Fig. 6.1 Ba shen fa *stretching*: neck, version 1, seated.

Clinical application and therapeutic effects

Where to apply the technique on the body

Ba shen fa can be applied to the cervical vertebrae of the neck, the lumbar vertebrae and most joints, especially the shoulders, elbows, wrists, fingers, toes and ankles. It can also be applied to the knees and the hips, but this can be hard work if you are working alone.

How to apply Ba shen fa

Ba shen fa gives space to the joints and helps the channel sinews that surround them to release. It is relatively straightforward to apply and involves stretching and extending the joints and their surrounding muscles, ligaments and tendons. Use it towards the end of treatment after the analgesic stage. Traction is created by holding either side of a joint and by pulling your hands in opposite directions, or in the case of Ba shen fa for the neck, you are using the patient's own body weight for the counter-traction. A few examples of how to apply Ba shen fa to different joints follow.

Applying Ba shen fa to the neck

There are three common ways to apply Ba shen fa to the cervical vertebrae of the neck. Practice them on all your fellow students and colleagues and you will probably find that you become particularly comfortable with one of them. It is very useful in practice to have the versatility of being able to apply one of the seated versions and the lying down supine version of Ba shen fa.

Seated position – version 1 Stand behind your seated patient with your feet shoulder width apart and knees slightly bent. Ground and center yourself. Hold your patient's head with your palms at the sides of their face around the area of the zygomatic arch and bring your thumbs to Fengchi GB20. Pressing with your thumbs into

GB20 and holding the sides of their face firmly, lift their head up, gradually creating traction to the cervical vertebrae until there is a natural resistance. Hold the traction for about 10–20 seconds and then slowly release.

Repeat this 2–3 times. In between each stretch, apply some Na fa, Rou fa or other technique to relax the neck muscles. (Fig. 6.1)

Seated position – version 2 For this version it is ideal to have your patient sitting on a low stool. Stand to one side of your seated patient, with your feet twice your own shoulder width apart and your knees bent, in a half squat position. Rest your patient's chin in the cubital crease of your flexed right elbow, holding their head securely between your upper arm and forearm. With your left hand, support the back of their head either with your palm at the occiput or by holding just under the occiput with an 'L' shape formed between your thumb and index finger. Keeping the balance between the back and front even, gradually begin to stand up from your half squat. Lift steadily and slowly in a controlled manner, stretching the neck until there is a natural resistance. Hold this traction for about 10–20 seconds and then gradually and slowly release, coming back into a half squat.

Repeat this 2–3 times, relaxing the neck muscles with basic or compound techniques. Anything based on Rou fa or Na fa does this job very well. (Fig. 6.2)

Lying down supine position Sit at the head of your patient who is lying down supine without a pillow under their head. Put one hand under the back of their head and hold the occiput. Cup their chin in the palm of your other hand. Keeping your arms straight, gradually lean back into your back, stretching their neck to create traction until there is a natural resistance. Hold the stretch for about 20 seconds then slowly release.

As before, repeat 2–3 times, relaxing the muscles in between each stretch.

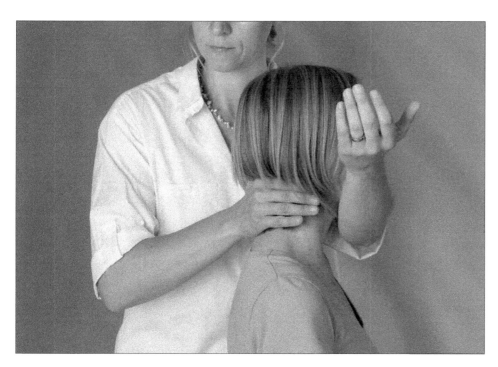

Fig. 6.2 Ba shen fa *stretching*: neck, version 2, seated.

Applying Ba shen fa to the lower back

There are two common methods of applying Ba shen fa to the lumbar vertebrae: the supine method which traditionally would have been applied with the help of an assistant and the back-to-back lifting method which is sometimes referred to as *Bei fa*.

Lying down supine position Stand at the feet of your patient who is lying down supine. Take hold of their lower legs just above the ankles and lift them up a little off the bench. If you are lucky enough to be working with a team of practitioners, in a pair or with an assistant, then ask them to hold under the patient's armpits so that they can fix the patient's upper body and provide some counter-traction. If you are working alone, ask your patient to take hold of the sides of the bench in order to keep their upper body steady while you apply the stretch.

Ask your patient to take some deep breaths into their belly. Working with their breath, slowly and steadily lean backwards, keeping your arms straight and using your body weight to gradually create the lumbar traction. With each exhalation, relax your body weight back a little more until there is a natural resistance. Hold the stretch for about 30 seconds, then gradually release (Fig. 6.3). If you are working with an assistant they can either just stay put, fixing the armpits, or they can apply counter-traction by keeping their arms straight and leaning their body weight back.

Repeat 2–3 times. Try using Dou fa in between each stretch to release the hips.

Back-to-back lifting This variation of Ba shen fa, or Bei fa as it is sometimes called, can only be performed on patients who are about the same height and weight as you are, or smaller and lighter. Do not even think about it if your patient is heavier and or taller than you are, or if you have any back problems yourself.

Stand back to back with the patient, with your feet shoulder width apart and link arms with your patient.

Ask your patient to relax and to breathe deeply into their abdomen. On the patient's out breath, bend forward from your waist, bending your knees slightly and lifting the patient off the floor to produce a hyperextension of the lumbar vertebrae and the extensor muscles of the Bladder channel sinew. The back of your patient's head should be relaxed at the level of your nape and their waist supported by your hips.

While the patient is suspended on your back, ask them to relax as much as possible, continuing to breathe deeply into any tension that they feel. To add to the stretch and for further release of the muscles, alternate rhythmically between straightening and bending your knees. When your legs are straight, try and gently shake the patient using your hips. After about a minute, gradually come up, releasing the patient back to the floor. If at any time you or your patient feels any pain then come back up.

You can repeat this stretch several times. Try using Pai fa on your patient's lumbar muscles in between stretches.

Applying Ba shen fa to the shoulder

There are several methods of stretching the shoulder. The three most common versions follow.

Straightforward shoulder traction in a seated position With your patient seated, stand behind and to the side of the shoulder you want to stretch. Hold the shoulder just proximal to the joint with one hand and apply some pressure. Hold the forearm just above the wrist with your other hand, gradually raise the patient's arm to 90 degrees and then stretch by keeping the pressure at the top of the shoulder and pulling away with the hand that holds the forearm. Lean your body weight in the direction of the stretch to help the traction and keep stretching gradually and smoothly until you feel a natural resistance.

Hold the stretch for 10–30 seconds. Encourage the patient to use their breath to help to release feelings of stiffness, restriction and discomfort. To encourage further

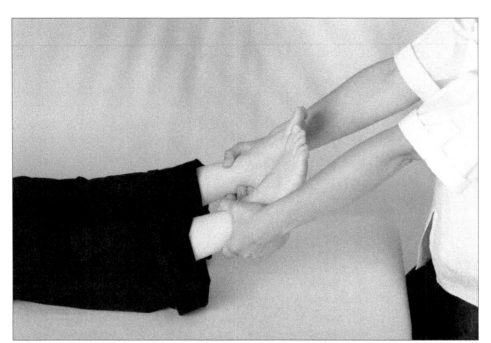

Fig. 6.3 Ba shen fa *stretching*: lower back, patient supine.

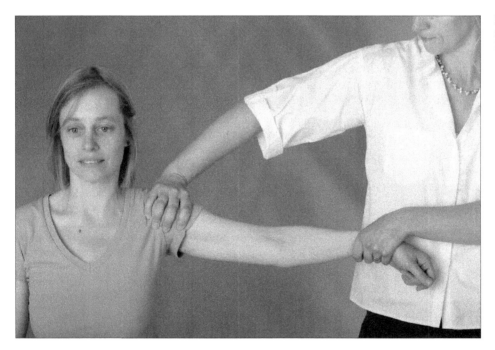

Fig. 6.4 Ba shen fa *stretching*: straightforward shoulder traction in a seated position.

release of the sinews and joint, sway or gently rock the arm back and forth during the stretch. (Fig. 6.4)

Shoulder traction with the patient's arm over your shoulder With your patient seated, kneel down on one knee to the side you want to stretch. Put your patient's arm over your shoulder. With interlaced fingers, hold the patient's shoulder with both hands. Apply Ya fa suppression to the shoulder and at the same time gradually raise yourself up from the kneeling position creating a stretch, then lower yourself back down. Work gradually, moving up and down, rising a little more with each stretch, until you come to the place of natural resistance.

Hold the stretch for 10–20 seconds and then release. Because you are using the leverage of your own body, there is very little effort required on your part. This is particularly useful if you have a patient who is much bigger and heavier than you are. If you rock your body gently from side to side during the stretch, this will produce further release of the joint and surrounding muscles.

In between stretches, try applying some Rou fa to the shoulder, keep your fingers interlaced and use the heels of your palms. Cuo fa is another useful technique to use between stretches. (Fig. 6.5)

Shoulder traction with the patient supine This method is similar to straightforward seated traction. With your

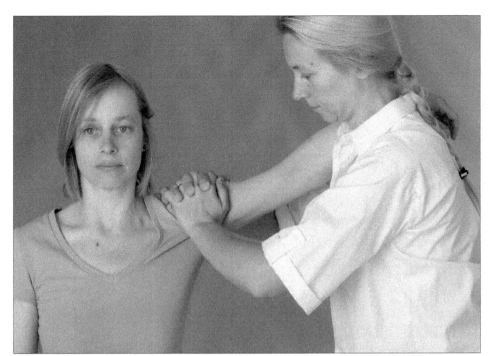

Fig. 6.5 Ba shen fa *stretching*: shoulder traction with the patient's arm over your shoulder.

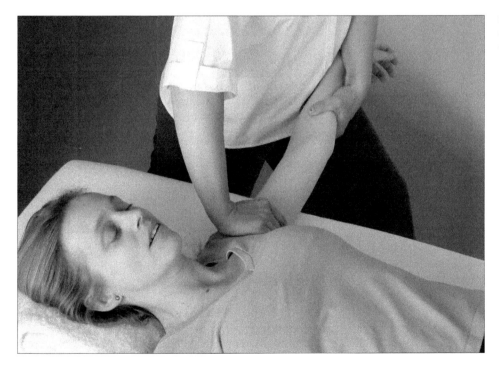

Fig. 6.6 Ba shen fa *stretching*: shoulder traction with the patient supine.

patient lying down supine, abduct their arm, holding either the top or the anterior aspect of the shoulder with one hand and their forearm with your other hand. Fix the shoulder and gradually pull the forearm to create traction. Hold for about 20 seconds and then release. (Fig. 6.6)

Repeat a few times. Try combining this variation of Ba shen fa with compound technique pinching–grasping applied to the Zhongfu LU1, Yunmen LU2 area.

Generally, to apply Ba shen fa to the joints of the wrist, ankle, knee, elbow, fingers and toes, hold either side of the joint you want to stretch and steadily and evenly pull your hands in opposite directions, hold the traction as before and gradually release.

Applying Ba shen fa to the elbow

Other than the general method mentioned above, there is another useful version of Ba shen fa for the elbow. With your patient either sitting or lying supine, flex their elbow and hold it underneath with one hand. Take hold of their forearm just above the wrist with your

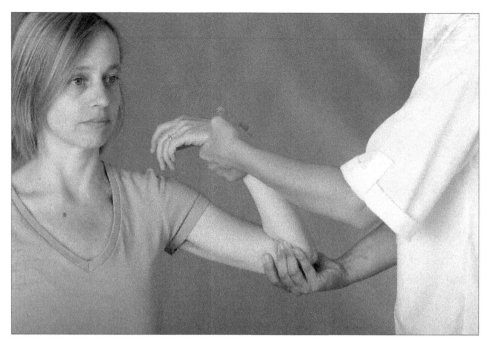

Fig. 6.7 Ba shen fa *stretching*: to the elbow.

other hand and lean your body weight backwards to create the traction. (Fig. 6.7)

Therapeutic effects

Ba shen fa is used to create space in the joints, allowing Qi and Blood to flow freely and providing the necessary nourishment and lubrication that joints require for comfortable, unrestricted and painless movement within their appropriate and natural range. It relaxes muscles and tendons, frees obstructions from the joints and channel sinews, releases adhesions, helps to realign the joints and alleviates pain.

Common uses

Ba shen fa is mainly used to treat Bi syndrome, Wei syndrome and muscular skeletal problems and injuries such as frozen shoulder, tennis elbow, acute lumbar sprain, displaced joints, repetitive strain injury (RSI), carpal tunnel syndrome, trigger finger, general stiffness of the muscles, tendons and ligaments.

When applied to the neck it is very useful as part of treatment for headaches and migraine.

Tips for practice

- Use Ba shen fa towards the end of treatment. Relax, warm and dredge the relevant channel sinews with other techniques first.
- The traction applied is increased gradually and evenly, avoiding any sudden rough movements.
- Hold the stretch for long enough for it to be therapeutically effective: 20–30 seconds is ideal.
- This technique must be applied with great care to articular deformity and rigidity.

Yao fa *rotating*

Yao fa is a passive circular movement that involves the smooth rotation of a joint within its natural range of movement. It is mainly used in the treatment of muscular skeletal ailments to bring Qi and Blood to the joints to lubricate them and to relax the muscles and tendons.

Clinical application and therapeutic effects

Where to apply the technique on the body

Yao fa can be applied to any joint in the body; in practice it is most commonly applied to the neck, shoulders, elbows, wrists, ankles, hips, fingers and toes.

How to apply Yao fa

Apply Yao fa either towards the end of treatment when the channel sinews are warm and relaxed and any relevant points have been stimulated, or in the analgesic phase where you can apply Yao fa between other techniques. In practice, Yao fa coordinates well with other basic and compound techniques, particularly An fa, Rou fa, Na fa and the compound versions of these.

Some patients find it difficult to relax and to give you the weight of their arm, leg or head. This in itself provides some interesting information about their ability to trust and let go. If this is the case, help them to become aware of it and encourage them to relax and let go. Reassure them and apply Yao fa with confidence, gently but firmly. Asking your patient to breathe into any areas of tension or discomfort is very helpful.

Below are descriptions of how to apply the versions of Yao fa that will be the most useful to you in practice.

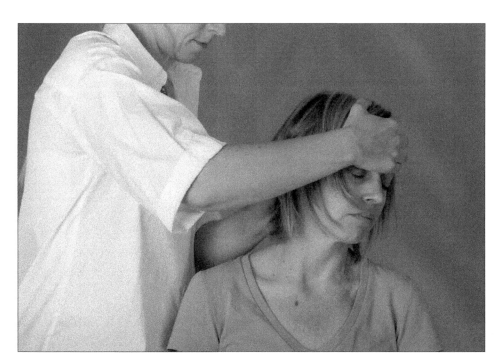

Fig. 6.8 Yao fa *rotating*: neck.

Applying Yao fa to the neck

With your patient seated, stand behind and slightly to one side of them. Relax, ground and center yourself. There are two ways of holding the head: either hold with one hand under the chin and the other on top of the head, or hold with one hand holding the forehead and the other holding the occiput. Try both ways and settle on whichever method feels more natural to you.

Starting with small circles, begin to rotate your patient's head slowly and smoothly in either a clockwise or anti-clockwise direction. Gradually increase the range of the rotation, always keeping it smooth and controlled with no sudden jerky movements. Imagine you are holding a football in your hands and are rolling it around between your palms. Try to let the rotation movement start from your Dantian; use your body to help to create the motion rather than just rotating with your arms.

Rotate about 10 times in one direction and then repeat rotating the other way. (Fig 6.8)

Applying Yao fa to the shoulder, with the patient seated

There are several variations of seated shoulder Yao fa. The three most common and clinically useful follow.

1. Straightforward Stand to the side of your patient behind their shoulder with your feet apart and one foot in front of the other. This position allows you to rock your body weight back and forth between your front and back foot to help create an effortless rotation on your part. Take hold of your patient's arm with one hand by holding either their forearm just above the wrist, or by supporting underneath their elbow. Raise their arm to the side to roughly shoulder level. Hold the top of their shoulder firmly with your other hand and begin to rotate either forwards or backwards. Start with small circles working slowly and smoothly. Gradually increase the

amplitude of the rotation by using your body to rock forward as you bring the arm up and around into forward extension, rocking back as you bring the arm down and into backward extension.

If the joint is very restricted, try applying An fa to one of the major points around the shoulder such as Jianyu LI15 while you are performing Yao fa. You will find that you can increase the amplitude much further as the use of An fa allows further release of the restricted joint and surrounding muscles.

If you are supporting the elbow, try applying An fa to Quchi LI11. Be creative and experiment by coordinating Yao fa with other techniques. For example, try applying kneading–grasping and the other compound versions of Na fa to the shoulder muscles while you rotate. (Fig. 6.9)

2. Yao fa with a large amplitude This is very similar to the above method. Stand to the side of your patient in front of their shoulder. Hold their arm just above the wrist with one hand and hold their shoulder with the other. Take a large step forward as you rotate their arm up and into forward extension and then step back as you bring their arm down and into backward extension.

The idea of this version is that you take the joint to the end of its natural full range of movement by rotating with the largest possible amplitude.

3. Yao fa with a flexed elbow and supported forearm This is a gentle version of Yao fa that circumflexes the shoulder joint and is useful if there is a lot of restriction or if the patient is finding it difficult to let go. Standing to the right side of your patient with your right foot in front of your left, hold their right shoulder with your left hand. Flex their elbow and rest the anterior aspect of their pronated right forearm on the anterior aspect of your supinated right forearm; their elbow is resting in your cubital crease. Hold onto their shoulder firmly and circle their arm using your body to rock forward and back.

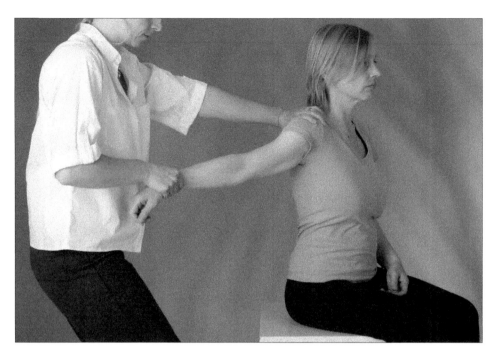

Fig. 6.9 Yao fa *rotating*: shoulder, version 1.

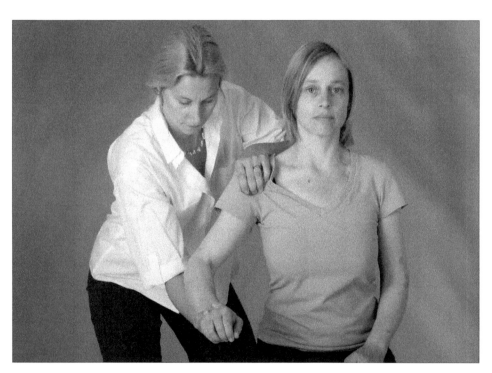

Fig. 6.10 Yao fa *rotating*: shoulder, version 3.

Circle several times in both directions. Swap sides and repeat. (Fig. 6.10)

Applying Yao fa to the shoulder, with the patient lying down prone

I use this method a lot in practice as it is excellent for helping to release the rhomboids and trapezius muscles and the Tai Yang channel sinews.

If you are working on your patient's right shoulder, stand to their right and take hold of their right forearm with your left hand and extend their arm backwards. Thread your right arm under their right elbow and bring your palm to their scapula with your fingers flexed and press into the suprascapular fossar. Rocking your body weight back and forth, circle their scapula and pull their forearm. Try it in both directions and on both shoulders.

This version of Yao fa brings the scapula through the movements of elevation, retraction, depression and protraction. (Fig. 6.11)

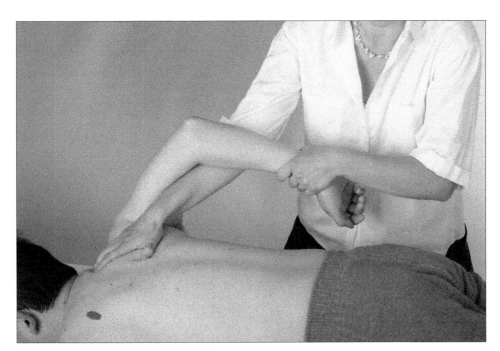

Fig. 6.11 Yao fa *rotating*: shoulder, patient prone.

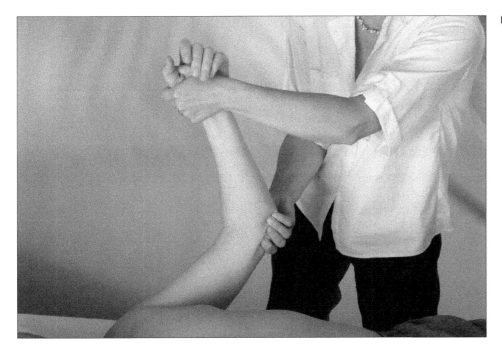

Fig. 6.12 Yao fa: to elbow.

Applying Yao fa to the elbow

Stand to one side of your patient and take hold of their flexed elbow with one hand, pressing LI11 with your thumb and Shaohai HT3 with your middle finger. Hold their wrist with your other hand and begin to circle the forearm clockwise and then anti-clockwise, starting with small circles and gradually increasing the range of the movement. (Fig. 6.12)

Applying Yao fa to the wrist

There are two variations of wrist Yao fa. The simplest method is to hold the patient's forearm just above the wrist with one hand and their fingers with your other hand. Rotate their wrist joint gently, clockwise and anti-clockwise several times in each direction. (Fig. 6.13)

Another method that I find useful is to hold the patient's hand with both of your hands, fingers underneath their palm and thumbs on top. Rotate the wrist by creating a rolling circular movement between your hands.

Applying Yao fa to the hip

Stand to the right-hand side of your patient who is lying down supine. Flex their right knee, bending it up towards

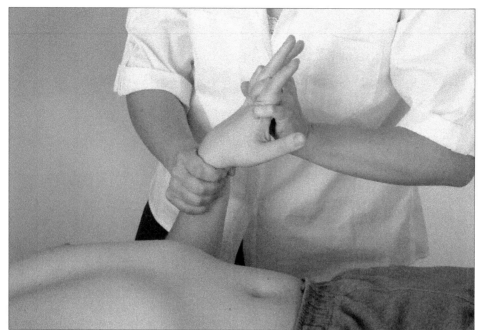

Fig. 6.13 Yao fa: to wrist.

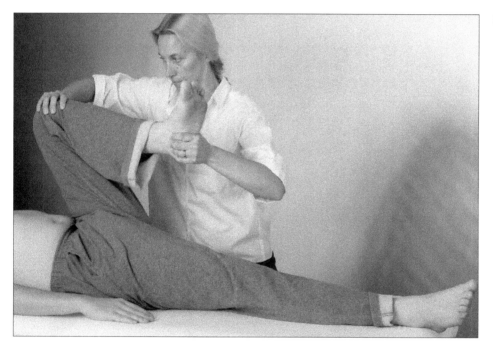

Fig. 6.14 Yao fa: to hip.

their chest. Take hold of either their right ankle or heel with your right hand and put your left hand either on top of or underneath their knee. Begin to rotate their hip in small smooth circles either clockwise or anti-clockwise. Let the movement come from your center, using your body rather than just the strength of your arms to create the rotation. As the hip begins to release, gradually increase the size of the rotation, feeling for any restriction and holding as you work. If the patient is able to, take their hip through its full rotational range of movement. Rotate several times in both directions. Repeat on the other side.

Patients often find it difficult to let themselves completely relax and let go during passive hip rotation, so it is important that you hold firmly and securely so that they feel as safe as possible. Encourage them to breathe deeply and to bring their attention to any areas of holding. (Fig. 6.14)

Applying Yao fa to the ankle

With your patient lying on their back, hold their heel with one hand and their toes with the other; rotate their foot several times in both directions. (Fig. 6.15)

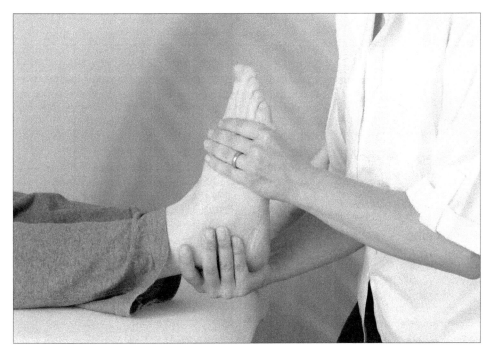

Fig. 6.15 Yao fa: to ankle.

Tips for practice

- Start with small circles and gradually and smoothly increase the rotation from narrow to wide.
- Always work on the good side as well as the problem side.
- Hold the patient softly but firmly so that they feel secure.
- Feel for any restriction, holding and tightness as you work.
- Do not force it or rush it.
- Work with the patient's breath and attention.

Therapeutic effects

Yao fa is used to lubricate the joints, helping Qi and Blood to flow to them and restoring the joints' full range of movement. It relaxes the muscles, tendons and ligaments, breaks up adhesions, and softens and releases muscular spasm.

Common uses

Yao fa is commonly used to treat both joint and channel sinew problems such as stiffness, swelling and pain of the joints and restricted joint mobility, frozen shoulder, tennis and golfer's elbow, injuries to muscles, tendons and ligaments, Bi syndrome and Wei syndrome.

Use Yao fa when Qi and Blood are stagnant and the channels are obstructed, and when Qi and Blood are insufficient and the channel sinews and joints are undernourished.

Ban fa *pulling–twisting*

Clinical application and therapeutic effects

Ban fa was traditionally part of bone-setting Tui na and was used as a major part of treatment for problems that came from injuries and traumas such as dislocated joints, displaced vertebrae and prolapsed discs. Tui na doctors became specialists in these joint manipulations after years of training and clinical experience and were the first port of call for patients with this type of injury. Even today, many people in China will seek out the Tui na departments of the TCM hospitals for treatment of these injuries rather than the treatment available in the hospitals of Western medicine.

In the West there is a big difference – people do not usually come to Tui na practitioners as their first port of call for treatment of acute injury and trauma. They are more likely to go to the hospital, to an osteopath or a chiropractor.

I am not an advocate of using Ban fa for overstretches and forced adjustments. I prefer to use it to stretch the channel sinews and to remind the joints of their full potential range of movements, creating deep passive stretches that often produce natural adjustments.

Several osteopaths that I have spoken to work with passive movements in this way and rarely if ever use forced adjustments. I have discussed this with several colleagues and fellow practitioners and the consensus of opinion is that far better results are achieved in the long run with muscular skeletal problems if we work on the channel sinews rather than attempting to force joints to adjust.

There are many different versions and varieties of Ban fa. Several of the most useful methods are described below.

Where to apply the technique on the body

Ban fa is most commonly applied to the neck, back and shoulders.

Applying Ban fa to the neck

I am not fond of the application of Ban fa on the neck. Personally I think it is unnecessary and that other methods can be used. I have included it here as it is used classically to reposition joints.

Either of the two versions below can be applied as assisted stretches without the final overstretch. In this case apply three times in both directions working with the patient's breath and holding the stretch for about 10 seconds.

Seated version With your patient sitting up straight, hold their forehead or the side of their head with one hand and their occiput with the other. Flex their head forward slightly by about 30 degrees. Laterally rotate their head to the maximum extent, until you feel a natural resistance. If you really feel it is necessary and you are completely confident in your application of the techniques, apply a momentary extra twist with a tiny amount of force by pulling your two hands in opposite directions. (Fig. 6.16)

Supine version With your patient lying down supine, put one hand under their occiput and hold their chin with your other hand. Create a little traction with the hand holding the occiput and then twist to one side until you are at the end of the range of movement and feel a natural resistance. At this point you can give a quick extra twist using a tiny amount of force.

Applying Ban fa to the shoulder

Forward flexion and backward extension With your patient sitting up straight, stand to their right-hand side and hold their right shoulder with your left hand. Hold their elbow with your right hand and slowly extend their

right arm forwards and then backwards to the end of the natural range of the movements. You can apply this simply as a stretch, repeating it three times, gradually increasing the stretch as you go. Or you can, after the third stretch, create an overstretch with a small swift movement, pulling the elbow in the direction of forward or backward extension while your right hand pushes the shoulder in the opposite direction. (Fig. 6.17)

Adduction version Your patient sits up straight as above, with their hands in front of their chest.

Standing close to their back, support their right shoulder with your right hand and grasp their right elbow with your left hand. Push their right shoulder forwards and pull their elbow inwards across their body. Stretch to the maximum degree and hold it for 10–20 seconds. Repeat three times, increasing the stretch with each repetition. Repeat on the other side. (Fig. 6.18)

Applying Ban fa to affect the sternocostal and mid-thoracic areas

Three common versions are described below.

Version 1 With your patient sitting on a stool or a low-backed chair, arms down by their sides, stand behind them and put your bent knee up against their mid-thoracic spine, directing your knee to the area you want to work on. Rest your foot on a stool or a convenient place at the back of the chair/stool that your patient is sitting on. Hold your patient's shoulders with your hands and pull them back towards you slowly and steadily to create a gentle to moderate stretch for the chest and mid-thoracic area of the back.

Version 2 The patient is seated as above but with their hands behind their head, fingers interlaced. Place your knee against the mid-thoracic spine or just to one side of the spine and hold their elbows with your hands. Ask your patient to breathe in, and on their out breath, pull their elbows back towards you and apply a little forward

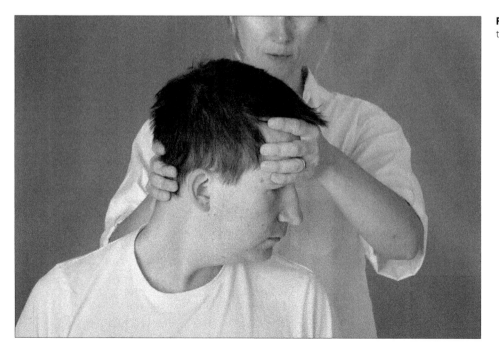

Fig. 6.16 Ban fa *pulling–twisting:* the neck, seated.

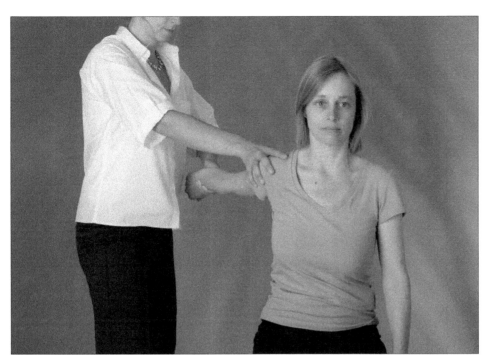

Fig. 6.17 Ban fa: on shoulder forward and backward extension.

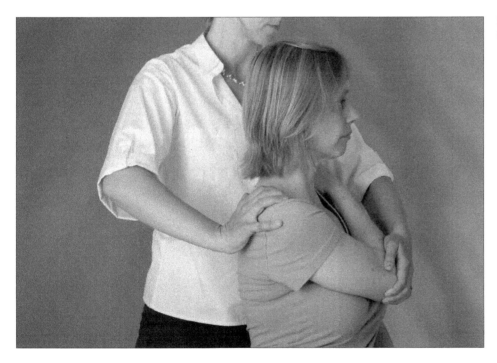

Fig. 6.18 Ban fa: on shoulder adduction.

pressure with your knee. On the patient's inhalation, push their elbows forward, rounding their upper back. Repeat this flexion and extension three times. (Fig. 6.19)
Version 3 This is very similar to version 2: your knee is to one side of the mid-thoracic spine and the patient's hands are behind their head with fingers interlaced as above. Bring your forearms under their armpits and in front of their upper arms. Now wind your forearms behind your patient's forearms and hold them just above their wrists. Working with your patient's breath, ask them to inhale and bend them forward a little, then on their

exhalation, pull them back, pressing forwards onto the vertebrae you want to affect. Classically, this version is used to correct displaced thoracic vertebrae. (Fig. 6.20)

Applying Ban fa to affect the lumbar and lower thoracic areas

Four main versions are used: supine, lateral, sitting and prone.
Supine twist With your patient lying down supine, stand to their left-hand side. Bend their left knee so that the

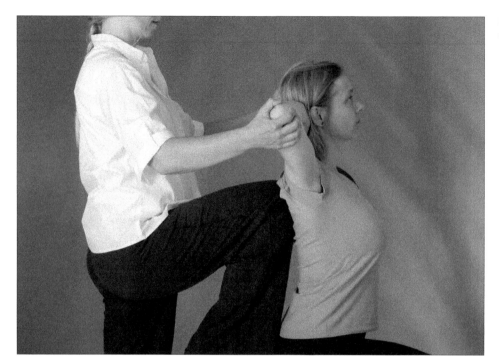

Fig. 6.19 Ban fa: sternocostal and mid-thoracic area, version 2.

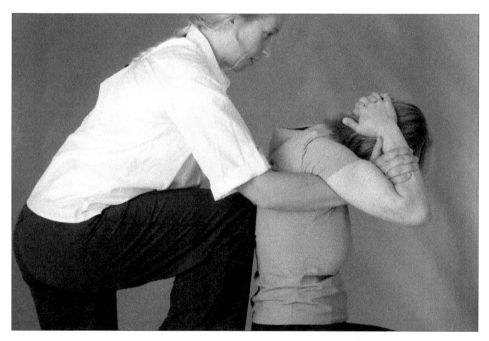

Fig. 6.20 Ban fa: sternocostal and mid-thoracic area, version 3.

heel is level with their right knee. Hold their left shoulder with your right hand or forearm and either hold their knee with your left hand or use your left forearm on the lateral side of the thigh. Keeping their left shoulder down by applying some pressure with your right palm or forearm, ask your patient to breathe in, and on their exhalation, push their left leg over their right to create the spinal twist. Take this twisting stretch to the natural end of the patient's range of movement. They should feel a stretch in the upper lumbar and/or the lower thoracic area and possibly the Gallbladder channel sinew at the hip. Hold the stretch for around 10–30 seconds and then

bring the patient back to lying on their back. Repeat this three times on both sides. You may hear a crack as you twist the patient's spine.

Lateral twist The lateral twist mainly affects the lumbar and lower thoracic area. It has a powerful effect on the Gallbladder channel and is useful in the treatment of liver pathology and Gallbladder channel sinew problems such as hip pain.

The key with this twist is to get the patient in the right position at the beginning.

Version 1 Stand behind your patient who is lying on their left side. Their left leg should be straight and their right

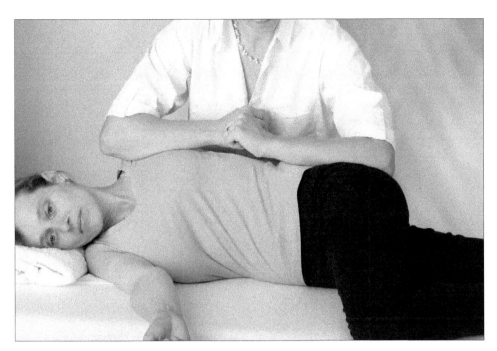

Fig. 6.21 Ban fa: lower thoracic and lumbar area.

leg bent. Ask your patient to breathe in, and then on their exhalation, simultaneously pull their right shoulder towards you and push their right hip away from you using either your hands or your forearms. Gradually take the stretch as far as you can within the patient's range of movement.

Ask your patient if they feel okay with the stretch and to let you know if they feel any pain. They should feel a stretch but no pain. If they feel pain then stop and work in a different way. If they are okay then hold the stretch for 10–30 seconds and then gently release the stretch and repeat this three times.

If you feel that it is safe, and only if you feel that therapeutically it will make a significant positive difference to treatment, then at the end of the stretch you can create an overstretch by pulling the shoulder back and pushing the hip forward with a small, quick and controlled forced thrust of both your hands or forearms. Sometimes during the stretch you will find that the back cracks quite naturally without any force. Always repeat on both sides. (Fig. 6.21)

Version 2 Stand in front of your patient who should be lying quite close to the edge of the treatment couch. The left leg should be straight and the right leg bent so that it comes down over the edge of the couch. Their left arm should be pulled out slightly from underneath them so that their scapula moves towards the couch. Tilt the patient's head back about 25 degrees, and then using your hands or forearms as above, pull the hip towards you and push the shoulder away. Then follow the above instructions for the stretch and the overstretch. (Fig. 6.22)

Seated lumbar twist With your patient seated, stand to their left side, facing them. Steady and block their legs with your own in order to keep their hips straight during the twist. Take hold of their left shoulder with your left hand and their right shoulder with your right hand. Turning from your waist, twist them towards you to the end of the natural range of movement and hold the twist for about 10–20 seconds and then release. Do this three times and then repeat on the other side. (Fig. 6.23)

Prone twist lifting the shoulder Your patient is lying down prone with their arms down by their sides. Stand to their right-hand side. Apply Ya fa *suppression* with your left palm over the spine at the level of Mingmen Du4 and lift their left shoulder with your right hand. Stretch the shoulder backwards gradually to create a spinal twist. Stretch the shoulder back as far as is comfortable for the patient; hold the twist for about 10 seconds and then release. You can work up the back with Ya fa moving up the spine a little with each twist. Apply to both sides. (Fig. 6.24)

Prone stretch lifting the leg Adjust your treatment couch quite low for this technique. The patient is lying down prone. Stand to their left. With your left hand, apply Ya fa using either your palm over Du4 or the heel of your palm to one side of the spine around the level of L2 to L5. Bring your right hand around and underneath their left thigh, holding just above the knee. Then while suppressing the lumbar area, simultaneously lift the left leg up extending it backwards. Slowly take the stretch to the end of the natural range of movement, if the patient is comfortable with it, and hold the stretch for about 10 seconds. Repeat this three times, increasing the stretch a little more each time. You can also rotate and rock the leg from side to side during the stretch to create further release of the lumbar and hip muscles.

This version of Ban fa can be used to correct deviated lumbar vertebrae. In this case, An fa is applied to the side of the affected vertebrae while the leg on the deviated side is extended backwards to the end of the range of movement. At this point a final thrust is performed between the two hands by lifting the leg with a quick overextension at the same time as applying additional pressure to the deviated vertebrae. (Fig. 6.25)

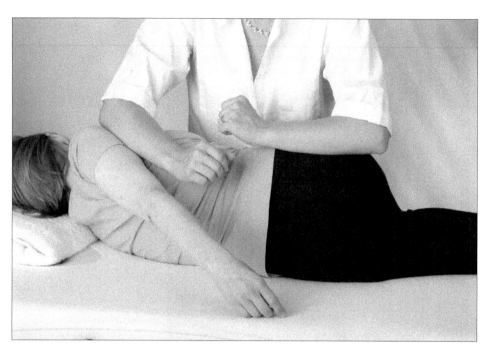

Fig. 6.22 Ban fa: lower thoracic and lumbar area, lateral twist, version 2.

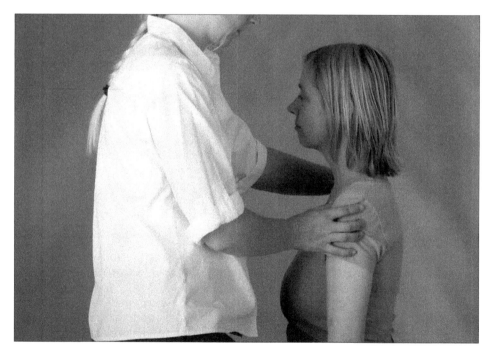

Fig. 6.23 Ban fa: lower thoracic and lumbar area, seated lumbar twist.

Therapeutic effects

Ban fa is used to relax muscular spasm and release adhesions, to bring Qi and Blood to the joints and their surrounding muscles, tendons and ligaments, and it helps to restore a joint's full articular range of movement. It moves Qi stagnation and Blood stasis and clears obstructions from the channels.

Common uses

Ban fa on the back is very effective for muscular/channel sinew problems affecting especially the Gallbladder and Bladder channel sinews. It can be very useful in the treatment of injuries such as lumbar sprain, adhesion and restriction to, for example, the greater psoas and sacrospinal muscles and the anterior and posterior longitudinal ligaments. It is useful for Wind-Damp-Cold Bi syndrome and Kidney-Qi Xu causing lower backache. The twists are also useful as part of treatment for Liver pathologies such as Liver-Qi stagnation and rebellious Liver-Qi invading the Stomach and Spleen. It is also classically used in the treatment of prolapsed lumbar discs.

Applied to the upper thoracic and the sternocostal area, Ban fa can be used to open the chest, helping with

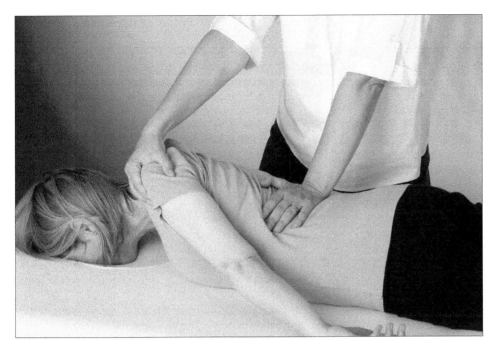

Fig. 6.24 Ban fa: lower thoracic and lumbar area, prone twist lifting the shoulder.

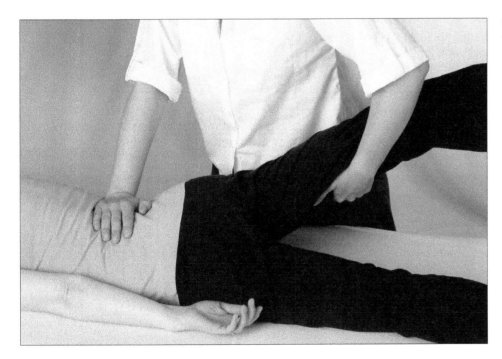

Fig. 6.25 Ban fa: lower thoracic and lumbar area, prone stretch lifting the leg.

problems related to Qi stagnation in the chest such as the characteristic stuffy, uncomfortable feeling in the chest often accompanied by irritability and/or depression. It is very useful for helping to balance the relationship between the pectoral muscles and the rhomboids; problems here can be a reflection of disharmony between the Lungs and the Liver. It is classically used to correct the position of displaced thoracic vertebrae.

Ban fa is usually applied to the shoulder for muscular and joint problems such as frozen shoulder, Bi syndrome and general restriction of the channel's sinews around the shoulder joint causing stiffness and compromised move-

ment of the shoulder. Classically, it would have been used for dislocation of the shoulder.

Neck Ban fa was classically used for bone setting and repositioning the joints.

General tips and contraindications for passive movements

Before applying a passive movement to a joint, first ask your patient to move the joint as far as possible through its natural range of movement, telling you when they

Tips for practice

- Use Ban fa at the end of treatment after lots of general work with other techniques to warm and relax the patient.
- Apply Ba shen fa and Yao fa before Ban fa. If these techniques are comfortable for the patient then proceed with Ban fa.
- **Do not** apply overstretches or forced thrusts until you have spent a lot of time applying the above techniques as assisted end-of-range stretches to lots of different people.
- Become clearly aware of the sensation of the body's natural resistance.
- Use the patient's breath when applying as end-of-range stretches.
- When using any of the twists or stretches, the movements should build up progressively.
- If performing the final overstretch, the movement should be quick and firm but not rough, and within the intended limits of the joint.
- **If in doubt, leave it out.**

feel restriction or pain. It is good practice to do this before and after treatment as it gives both you and your patient a means of assessing improvement and progress.

Before applying passive movements, stimulate distal and local points and work with basic, compound and coordinated techniques on the channel sinews that relate to the affected joint first. This will stimulate the flow of Qi and Blood, relax the muscles, tendons and ligaments and enable you to work on the joint safely and easily.

Yao fa and Ba shen fa are relatively simple and safe to perform; just remember to manipulate slowly and smoothly, stopping if you feel any resistance to what should be a normal movement.

If a patient is very elderly or frail and weak, only apply very gentle Yao fa or rocking movements to the joints but no other passive movements.

Contraindications

Do not apply any passive movements in the following circumstances:

- If you suspect that a joint is dislocated or that a bone is fractured
- To patients with cancer of the bone or if you suspect secondary bone cancer
- If you feel at all uncomfortable or worried about applying them

Do not apply any forced Ban fa manipulations to patients with:

- Hypertension – high blood pressure
- Hypotension – low blood pressure
- Heart disease
- Osteoporosis
- Spondylosis
- Ménière's disease
- Meningitis

Remember, if in doubt, leave it out! Seek the advice of a more experienced practitioner or colleague.

CHAPTER 7

Area foundation routines

Area foundation routines have two important purposes. They provide you with a structure for learning to develop your Tui na skills and with a framework for creating Tui na treatments.

A structure for developing your Tui na skills

Practicing the area foundation routines will help you to develop your techniques and to learn how to adapt them to different parts of the body. They bring together a logical sequence of techniques that move through the adaptive, analgesic and dissipative stages of treatment.

I suggest that you learn them like a dance routine until one technique flows smoothly into the next and they feel like second nature. If you do, your confidence will grow and you will become fluid and coordinated in your application.

Once the sequences are second nature, you can concentrate on other aspects of your practice such as relaxation and softness, bringing Qi to your hands, developing sensitivity and directing your attention.

A framework for creating treatments

One of the most challenging aspects of Tui na is choosing what techniques to apply and where and how to apply them. The area foundation routines make this process more manageable by providing the foundations for creating and building up Tui na treatments. The routines provide a framework, which can be utilized and adapted. Techniques and points can be added or removed, and particular aspects of a routine can be focused on according to the requirements of treatment.

Note-taking is also made easier. Instead of writing down every single technique that you want to apply, which would be very time-consuming, you can refer to the area routines that you want to use and note what you focused on, added or removed. For example, you may say that you applied the chest routine, focusing on gentle Tui fa and Rou fa in the intercostal spaces.

Health maintenance treatments

You can provide excellent preventative and health maintenance Tui na treatments by linking the area foundation routines together and following the general principles of treatment on page 130.

There are several versions of area routines. This is because every experienced practitioner and teacher will have developed their own variations along with their style of practice.

In the rest of this chapter, I have provided foundation routines that will help you to develop a broad range of techniques and become familiar with working through the three stages of treatment. As you gain experience and develop your own style of practice, you can, if you wish, experiment with creating your own foundation routines. Just remember to follow the three stages of treatment.

The area foundation routines I describe are:

- The head and face
- The neck and nape
- The back
- The upper limb
- The lower limb
- The chest and hypochondrium
- The abdomen

Head and face

The head routine is applied with the patient seated.

The techniques applied to the head should be performed over a cotton Tui na cloth unless the patient has very short hair in which case you can apply them directly to the head.

1. Tui fa and Mo fa

Stand in front of your patient supporting the back of their head with one hand. Bring Qi to your other hand and apply Tui fa and then Mo fa from the anterior to the posterior hairline using your palm and fingers. Work the left side of the head first, then the right and finally the center. Start slowly and gradually increase your speed.

Alternate between these two techniques until the patient's head feels hot.

2. Rou fa

Stand behind your patient, interlace your fingers and apply Rou fa to Fengchi GB20 using the minor thenar eminence of both hands.

3. Compound technique: grabbing–grasping

Grab and grasp the five channels of the head, from the anterior to the posterior hairline, about 10 times.

4. Ma fa

Apply Ma fa with your thumbs from the temporal hairline in front of your patient's ears to the mastoid process. Work gradually backwards and forwards several times until the area feels hot.

5. Pai fa

Using a loose fist or the palm of your hand, apply Pai fa to Baihui Du20 10 times.

The face routine is applied with the patient lying supine.

1. Tui fa

Using the palms of your hands, apply Tui fa gently to stroke your patient's forehead and temple area.

Using your thumbs alternately, push from Yintang to Shangxing Du23.

2. Ma fa

Wipe back and forth with your thumbs in horizontal lines from the eyebrows to the anterior hairline.

3. Compound technique: pinching–grasping

Pinch and grasp the eyebrows between your thumbs and index fingers from medial to lateral three times.

4. Yi zhi chan tui fa

Apply moving Yi zhi chan tui fa in a figure-of-eight around the eyes 6–10 times.

5. Rou fa

Knead Yintang and Tai Yang with your middle fingers.

6. An fa, Rou fa and the compound technique, kneading–pinching

Stimulate Zanzhu BL2, Benshen GB13, Yangbai GB14, Sibai ST2, Juliao ST3, Daying ST5, Touwei ST8, Yingxiang LI20, Renzhong Du26 and Chengjiang Ren24 using An fa and Rou fa or kneading–pinching, until the points are warm and slightly sore.

7. Ma fa

Using your index and middle fingers, wipe back and forth briskly from LI20 to BL2 until the area is very warm.

8. Compound technique: pinching–grasping

Pinch and grasp along the jaw line from Ren24 to Jiache ST6 using both hands, three times.

9. Rou fa

Knead underneath the jaw with your fingertips and knead the masseter muscle with your major thenar eminence at the same time. Apply to each side three times.

Apply light, brisk Rou fa with your thenar eminence to the jaw, cheeks, temples and forehead until warm.

10. Compound technique: kneading–pinching

Knead and pinch the ears, then lift and pull both ears three times.

11. Gua fa

Gently scratch the scalp with the tips of your fingers and/or nails along the anterior hairline from left to right and right to left three or four times.

To finish

Warming palm

Finally, rub your hands together until scorching hot, and then bring them over your patient's eyes, ears or temples according to their presenting disharmony. (Refer to p. 135 using breath and visualization for more ideas.)

The foundation routine for the head and face has a soothing, relaxing effect, and in my experience, patients love it. It can be applied to calm the Shen, expel Wind, disperse obstructed Wei Qi, improve vision, clear the sinuses, alleviate pain, and facilitate and regulate the rising of clear Yang.

With the addition of appropriate distal work, work on the back, chest, abdomen, and so on, this routine provides a very useful basis for the treatment of problems such as:

- Headaches and migraine
- Insomnia
- Stress
- Anxiety/depression
- Ear, nose and throat (ENT) problems

- Common cold
- Sinusitis
- Allergic rhinitis
- Dizziness
- Facial paralysis
- Tinnitus
- Toothache

Neck and nape

The neck and nape routine is applied with the patient seated.

Adaptive level

1. Tui fa

Support your patient's forehead with your non-dominant hand and apply Tui fa with your dominant hand using the tips of your index, middle and ring fingers. Work in lines from Fengfu Du16 to Dazhui Du14, Tianzhu BL10 to Dazhu BL11 and then using both hands from Fengchi GB20 to Jianjing GB21. Apply each about 5–10 times.

2. Rou fa

Apply Rou fa along the same lines as Tui fa above using your thenar muscle 3–5 times. Then using your thumb apply Rou fa between each of the cervical vertebrae, then just to one side of the vertebrae and then down the Bladder and Gallbladder channels of the neck.

Apply Rou fa with the heel of your palm all over the nape, top of the shoulders, scapula and the upper back until the muscles feel warm.

Analgesic level

3. Gun fa

Apply Gun fa all over the top of the shoulders, nape, the back and sides of the neck, incorporating some passive movements of the neck as you work. Apply for about 10 minutes.

4. Yi zhi chan tui fa, Ji fa, Zhen fa or An fa

Select a couple of local points to be stimulated, such as BL10, GB20, GB21, Jianzhongzhu SI15 and stimulate for 2–3 minutes using one or two of the above techniques.

5. Na fa

Knead and grasp the neck, from the occiput to the root of the nape several times. Pinch and grasp either side of the neck from BL10 to BL11 three times on each side. Knead and grasp gently along the sternocleidomastoid muscle three times on each side. Lift and grasp the top of both shoulders (GB21 area) briskly for about a minute.

6. Rou fa

Knead the patient's throat gently with the pads of your thumb and fingers several times, working along the sternocleidomastoid, the Stomach and Large Intestine channels.

Passive movements

7. Ba shen fa

Apply Ba shen fa to the neck three times remembering to work with your patient's breath. Apply kneading and grasping between each stretch.

8. Yao fa

Rotate the neck. Remember to start gently with small rotations and gradually increase the range of the movement. Do this in both directions.

Dissipative level

9. Pai fa, Ji dian fa and Ji fa

Apply loose fist Pai fa or five-finger Ji dian fa to the patient's neck and nape and Ji fa to the nape and top of both shoulders.

10. Whisking–sweeping

Whisk and sweep the nape, shoulders and upper back.

To finish

Warming palm

Finally, rub your hands together until scorching hot, and then bring them to the top of your patient's shoulders. (Refer to p. 135 using breath and visualization for more ideas.)

With the addition of appropriate distal and local points, this routine provides a useful basis for the treatment of problems such as:

- Restriction of neck movement, muscular tension, sprain, wry neck
- Cervical spondylosis
- Wind-Cold-Damp Bi syndrome
- Headache/migraine
- Insomnia
- Stress
- Anxiety/depression
- ENT problems
- Sore throat/hoarseness/vocal problems

Remember that for problems in the neck, you will need to work in the arm. Try applying the foundation routine for the upper limb before the neck and nape routine.

Back

The back routine is applied with the patient lying prone.

Adaptive level

1. Tui fa

Push with your palm along the Governing Vessel from Du14 to the coccyx. With both palms or the heels of your palms, move down the Bladder channel from the nape to the sacrum. With one palm, move across the Bladder channel pushing from the spine out to the sides of the body, working down gradually from the nape to the sacrum. Do each of these several times until the patient's back becomes warm.

2. Rou fa

Knead along the Governing Vessel and the Bladder channel from nape to sacrum with your whole palm or heel of your palm 3–5 times.

For variation, apply pinching–grasping or kneading–grasping to the top of the shoulder nearest to you and Rou fa along the Bladder channel on the opposite side.

Analgesic level

3. Gun fa

Apply Gun fa along the Bladder channel working up and down between the nape and the sacrum for about 10 minutes.

4. An fa/Ya fa and Rou fa

Press, suppress and knead with your thumbs or elbow along the Huatuojiaji points and the inner and outer lines of the Bladder channel from top to bottom. You can work the whole back or pick out particular points.

5. Ya fa

With one hand on top of the other and the power coming from both hands, suppress with your palms from the nape to the sacrum on either side of the spine. Work slowly, asking the patient to breathe slowly and deeply; let your hands follow their breath, suppressing with the patient's exhalation. This should feel soothing and relaxing.

Suppress the sacrum three times using the heel of your palm or forearm.

6. Rou fa

Apply Rou fa to the lower back, sacrum and buttocks using your forearms and the heels of your palms.

7. Tui fa

Using a little toasted sesame oil, dong qing gao or other suitable massage medium, apply Tui fa with your elbow from the nape to the sacrum, working just to one side of the spine along the line of the Huatuojiaji points 3 times on each side.

With one palm on top of the other, apply strong pushing with the heel of your palm from Shenshu BL23 to Zhibian BL54.

Dissipative level

8. Ji fa and Pai fa

Apply Ji fa and Pai fa from the nape to the sacrum either side of the spine. Apply Pai fa with a hollow palm over the spine.

9. Whisking–sweeping and Ji fa and Pai fa

Either alternate between whisking and sweeping and the striking techniques or use in combination as a coordinated technique working all over the back.

10. Ca fa

Apply Ca fa to the Bladder meridian either side of the spine, across the tops of the shoulders and across the lumbar and sacral areas using dong qing gao, woodlock oil or another suitable massage medium.

Passive movements

11. Ban fa

Apply supine or lateral twist Ban fa as an end-of-range stretch without force.

Supporting the kidneys

12. Rub your palms until scorching hot and place over Shenshu BL23. On your in breath, draw Qi in through Baihui Du20 into your Dantian, and on your out breath, release the Qi through Laogong PC8 into the patient's kidneys. Work like this for about 3 minutes.

Upper limb

The upper limb routine is applied with the patient seated.

Adaptive level

1. Tui fa

Push with your palm along the arm Yang and Yin channels from the shoulder to the hand, working with or against the flow of Qi depending on your diagnosis, until warm.

2. Rou fa

Knead with your palm or the heel of your palm, working gradually along the channels, Yang first and then Yin. Pay attention to the shoulder, elbow and wrist joints as you come to them.

3. Compound technique: holding–grasping

Hold and grasp 3–4 times from shoulder to wrist.

Analgesic level

4. Gun fa

Apply rolling to the shoulder joint and upper arm with one hand while the other hand supports the patient's arm and applies gentle rocking and twisting passive movements. Continue rolling gradually up and down the arm from shoulder to wrist focusing on the elbow joint when you come to it.

5. An rou fa

Press and knead with your thumb the major points around the shoulder, elbow and wrist such as Jianzhen

SI9, Tianzong SI11, Jianyu LI15, Jianliao TE14, Quchi LI11, Shousanli LI10, Chize L5, Xiaohai SI8, Waiguan SJ5, Neiguan PC6, Yangchi SJ4, Yangxi LI5 and Hegu LI4.

6. Compound versions of Na fa and Rou fa

Working along the Yang and Yin channels between the shoulder and the wrist, apply kneading–grasping, pinching–grasping, plucking–grasping, nipping–grasping and kneading–nipping. Work into fossas and points and places where channel sinews bind.

7. Nian fa and Rou fa

Apply holding and twisting to each finger three times and then Rou fa to the arm Yang channel Well points.

Dissipative level

8. Cuo fa

Rub roll the shoulder and then all the way down the arm three times then rub roll the palm.

9. Dou fa

Holding just above the wrist, apply Dou fa to the arm three times.

10. Pai fa, Ji dian fa and Ji fa

Apply loose fist and hollow palm Pai fa to the shoulder joint and up and down the Yang and Yin channels. Apply Ji dian fa around the joints and to areas of adhesion and holding. Apply Ji fa *chopping* between each of the patient's fingers.

Passive movements

11. Yao fa and Ba shen fa

Apply Yao fa and Ba shen fa to the shoulder, elbow, wrist and fingers.

12. Ban fa

Apply forward and backward extension Ban fa to the shoulder as a passive end-of-range movement stretch three times.

To finish

13. Ca fa

Using a massage medium such as woodlock oil, apply Ca fa to the shoulder joint using both hands on either side of the joint. Do the same with the elbow joint and then apply to the whole of the upper limb along the Yang and Yin channels.

14. Warming palm

Finally, rub your hands together until scorching hot, then hold a joint or another area that needs some support and Qi between your hands. (Refer to p. 135 for more ideas on using breath and visualization.)

Most of this area foundation routine could also be applied with your patient lying down supine. Make adjustments to the techniques according to the position.

This routine provides a framework that is useful to apply as either a way into treatment or as part of treatment for problems such as:

- Bi syndromes and traumas affecting the joints, muscles and tendons of the upper limb, for example frozen shoulder, tennis elbow, carpal tunnel syndrome, repetitive strain injury (RSI), cervical spondylosis, wry neck
- Chronic neck and shoulder tension
- Problems affecting the chest such as palpitations, chest Bi syndrome, cough and asthma
- Headaches and ENT problems

The upper limb can be used as a passageway for dredging and draining pathogenic factors and stagnant Qi from held emotions that are affecting the upper part of the body.

Lower limb

Begin the routine with the patient lying prone.

Adaptive level

1. Tui fa

Push with your palm along the Bladder and Gallbladder channels from the buttocks to the toes until warm.

2. Rou fa

Knead with your palm or the heel of your palm, working gradually along the Bladder and Gallbladder channels.

3. Compound technique: holding–grasping

Hold and grasp along the Bladder channel 3–4 times from the buttocks to the ankles.

Analgesic level

4. Gun fa

Apply Gun fa along the Bladder channel from the buttocks to the ankles. Work up and down the leg several times, increasing your depth and power gradually. You can also incorporate passive flexion and extension of the knee joint while applying Gun fa to the gluteal area.

5. Ya fa

Using your palm or the heel of your palm, apply Ya fa to the Bladder channel from the buttocks to the ankles. Then apply elbow Ya fa and Rou fa to Zhibian BL54, Huantiao GB30, Chengfu BL36, Yinmen BL37 and Chengshan BL57.

6. Compound technique: pushing–pressing

Using both thumbs, push and press Weizhong BL40.

7. Compound technique: kneading–grasping

Work along the Bladder and Gallbladder channels from the buttocks to the ankles with kneading–grasping. Work into fossas and points and places where the channel sinews bind.

Knead and grasp either side of the Achilles tendon to stimulate Kunlun BL60 and Taixi KD3.

8. Compound technique: pinching–grasping

Pinch and grasp along the Bladder channel from BL40 to Zhiyin BL67.

9. An fa

With your patient's lower leg supported either on your own thigh or on pillows, apply An fa to the heels and soles of the feet using your knuckles.

10. Ca fa

Scrub Yongquan KD1 with your knuckles until scorching hot.

11. Nian fa

Hold and twist each toe three times.

Dissipative level

12. Pai fa and Ji fa

Apply Pai fa or Ji fa from the buttocks to the ankles.

13. Compound technique: whisking–sweeping

Whisk and sweep briskly along the leg.

Now ask the patient to turn over so they are lying supine and continue.

Adaptive level

14. Tui fa and Rou fa

Push and knead along the Stomach channel and along the Spleen, Liver and Kidney channels until warm.

Analgesic level

15. Gun fa

Apply Gun fa to the Stomach channel working from Biguan ST31 to Jiexi ST41.

16. Compound technique: pinching–grasping

Pinch and grasp along the Stomach channel and along the Yin channels of the leg, focusing on major points along the way.

Dissipative level

17. Pai fa

Knock with your palm or a loose fist along the Stomach channel and the Yin channels of the leg.

18. Ca fa

Scrub along the Stomach channel and the Yin channels, focusing the technique around the medial and lateral sides of the knee.

Passive movements

19. Yao fa

Perform Yao fa on the hips and ankles.

20. Ba shen fa

Use Ba shen fa to extend the legs and stretch the joints. Hold the patient's ankles and raise both legs up simultaneously. Use your body weight to apply the stretch by leaning backwards. While maintaining a gentle stretch, swing the patient's legs from side to side and circle the legs clockwise then anti-clockwise a few times.

21. Duo fa

Holding the patient's ankle, perform Dou fa on each leg.

This foundation routine for the lower limb will help to lubricate the joints, relax and release the leg channel sinews, activate and invigorate the circulation of Qi and Blood, dredge and expel pathogenic factors and stop pain. It can provide a framework for treatment of various problems including:

- Bi syndromes such as osteoarthritis and rheumatoid arthritis
- Traumas affecting the joints, muscles and tendons of the lower limb
- Sciatica
- General muscle pain
- Atrophy of the leg muscles
- Back problems – working on the lower limb is essential

The lower limb can be used as a passageway for dredging and draining pathogens and stagnant Qi that are affecting the lower part of the body.

Chest and hypochondrium

The chest and hypochondrium routine is applied with the patient lying supine.

Adaptive level

1. Tui fa

Push with your palm across the chest from the sternum to the Zhongfu LU1, Yunmen LU2 area. Work one side then the other. Push from Tiantu Ren22, Shanzhong Ren17 using either the pads of three fingers or the heel of your palm. Push across the ribs with both palms working from the midline out.

2. Rou fa

Knead with your palm or the heel of your palm all over the chest, ribs and down the Yin channels of the arms.

Analgesic level

3. An fa, Rou fa and Ma fa

Press and knead Ren17 and LU1 with your thumb.

Press and knead the intercostal spaces with both of your thumbs, working from the midline out and working down to the level of the 3rd or 4th intercostal space, pressing and kneading each place several times. After pressing and kneading each intercostal space, apply Ma fa briskly back and forth.

4. Compound technique: kneading–grasping

With your thumb in the LU1 area and your fingers in the axilla, knead and grasp the lateral side of the greater pectoral muscle several times on both sides.

5. Compound technique: pushing–pressing

Apply pushing–pressing to the subclavicular fossa.

Dissipative level

6. Ji dian fa and Zhen fa

Apply light dotting to the chest along the Ren, Kidney and Stomach channels and in the LU1–2 area. Apply Zhen fa either with your middle finger or palm to two or three major points of the chest such as Ren17, Shufu KD27 and LU1.

7. Pai fa

Apply palm or loose fist knocking to the flanks and lower ribs.

8. Zhen fa

Apply palm Zhen fa to the lower ribs over the area of Qimen Liv14.

9. An fa to open the lungs

Put one hand on top of the other. Ask your patient to breathe in; on their out breath, press their chest with a pumping action, gradually increasing the pressure until they have completely exhaled. Release the pressure as your patient breathes in. Do this three times on the chest, and then repeat the same action on each side of the ribcage, encouraging your patient to expand their ribcage when they inhale.

10. Ca fa

Using an appropriate massage medium, scrub across the chest, along the flanks and across the lower ribs using either your minor thenar eminence or your palm.

11. Cuo fa

Ask your patient to sit up on the treatment couch. Apply rub rolling to their ribcage 3–5 times.

To finish

Warming palm

Rub your hands together until scorching hot and apply to points or areas of the chest or ribs that need the most support. (Refer to p. 135 for more ideas on using breath and visualization.)

The foundation routine for the chest and ribs soothes Liver-Qi, descends rebellious Qi, moves stagnation,

opens the chest, promotes expectoration of Phlegm, strengthens Lung-Qi, tonifies the Upper Jiao and the Sea of Qi of the chest, benefits the diaphragm and aids respiration and calms the Shen.

With the addition of appropriate distal work, work on the back, abdomen, head and so on, this routine provides a very useful basis for the treatment of problems such as:

- Chest pain
- Asthma
- Cough
- Palpitations
- Hypochondriac pain
- Epigastric pain
- Plum stone throat
- Migraine
- Irritable bowel syndrome (IBS)
- Premenstrual tension (PMT) and menstrual problems
- Insomnia
- Stress/depression/anxiety

Abdomen

The abdomen routine is applied with the patient lying supine.

Adaptive level

1. Tui fa

Push with both palms from just below the ribs to the upper border of the pubic bone. Imagine drawing a line with your Laogong PC8 along the patient's Stomach channel. Do this until the belly becomes warm.

Tui fa can be applied with one or both palms to any of the channels that move through the abdomen, pushing with or against the flow of Qi according to your treatment principle.

2. Mo fa

Round rub the abdomen with the palm of one hand 36 times clockwise then 36 times anti-clockwise to harmonize the digestion. If the patient is constipated, work in a clockwise direction. If they have diarrhea, work anti-clockwise.

3. Rou fa

Knead Zhongwan Ren12, Tianshu ST25 and Qihai Ren6 with the palm of your hand until warm.

Analgesic level

4. Local point stimulation with An fa and Rou fa or Yi zhi chan tui fa

Press and knead ST25 with your thumbs, working both points at the same time. Then apply Yi zhi chan tui fa, or An fa and Rou fa to Ren12, Zhangmen Liv13 or other suitable points according to your diagnosis. Stimulate each point for about 3 minutes.

5. Coordinated technique: forearm Rou fa and Gun fa

Apply forearm Rou fa to the abdomen, concentrating on the areas of Ren12 and Shenque Ren8, and Gun fa with your other hand along the Stomach channel of the leg.

6. Cat's paw An fa

Put the palms of both hands in a horizontal line across the abdomen at the level of the navel. Create a wave-like motion, pressing from the heel of your right palm through to the fingers and then passing the wave to the heel of your left palm. Imagine that you are gradually and smoothly rolling a ball that is inside the patient's abdomen from side to side. Think of a cat kneading a blanket. This motion helps to harmonize the intestines.

Dissipative level

7. Compound technique: lifting–grasping

Lift and grasp the abdomen, working along the channels. Lift and grasp and roll the flesh back and forth between your fingers or lift, grasp and jerk to the left and right and release.

8. Zhen fa

Vibrate with your right palm over the navel, ST25/Daheng SP15 and Ren6/Guanyuan Ren4.

9. Pai fa

Knock the abdomen with a cupped palm.

To finish

Warming palm

Rub your hands together until scorching hot and apply to points or areas of the abdomen that need the most support. (Refer to p. 135 using breath and visualization for more ideas.)

The abdominal routine strengthens the Spleen and Stomach, tonifies Qi, harmonizes the Stomach and Intestines, harmonizes the Middle Jiao, moves stagnation, warms the Kidneys, and regulates the function of the Ren and Chong Mai.

With the addition of appropriate distal work, and work on the back, chest and ribs, this routine provides a very useful basis for the treatment of problems such as:

- IBS
- Constipation
- Diarrhea
- Epigastric pain
- Abdominal pain
- Indigestion
- Poor appetite
- Belching and flatulence
- Painful periods
- Irregular menstruation
- Amenorrhea
- Fibroids
- PMT
- Infertility

CHAPTER **8**

Ancillary therapies

The ancillary therapies of cupping, gua sha and moxibustion are powerful and potent therapeutic methods that can be applied in conjunction with Tui na treatment to produce excellent results. In this chapter I will give a brief description of each of the three therapies, how to apply them, their therapeutic effects and some suggestions for when to use them. As with Tui na, these therapies are practical and need to be taught by an experienced practitioner.

You can refer to the recommended reading section at the end of this book for more detailed information.

Cupping

Cupping is an ancient therapy that has been used as part of folk medicine all over the world. The earliest recorded use of cupping is found in *A Handbook of Prescriptions for Emergencies* written by the famous Taoist alchemist and herbalist, Ge Hong (AD281–341). Cupping was used in English hospitals in the 1830s to treat contagious diseases; it was so popular at the time that there were paid 'cuppers' working in the hospitals. Originally, cups were made from animal horns, then pottery and bamboo. Today they are made out of thick glass.

Cupping is used to release the Exterior, and draw external pathogens up to the surface and out through the open pores. It stimulates and regulates the flow of Qi and Blood and can be used to relax the muscles, move stagnant Qi and Blood and ease pain.

How to apply cupping

To create the suction, which enables the cups to stick to the skin, you have to remove the oxygen from the cup by briefly putting a flame into it (Fig. 8.1).

To apply cupping:

1. Lubricate the patient's skin at the area you want to cup with a little base oil such as grapeseed oil.
2. Bring the cups that you want to use close to the patient.
3. Soak a small ball of cotton wool in surgical spirits and squeeze out any excess.
4. Hold the soaked ball of cotton wool with a pair of long-handled forceps in your dominant hand and light it.
5. Warm the rim of the glass cup with the flame so that it is not cold when you put it onto your patient's skin. Test the temperature of the cup rim on the back of your hand.
6. Holding the cup close to the area you want to apply it to, put the flame into the cup very briefly, then withdraw the flame and immediately apply the cup to the skin. If you hold the cup too far away from the skin, by the time you apply it, oxygen will have returned to the cup and there will be very little or no suction.
7. Keep the flame away from the patient. When you have finished cupping, either blow out the flame or put it in water to extinguish it.

8. To remove the cups, press the skin by the edge of the cup firmly with the fingers of one hand to allow air in and gently lift the cup off with the other hand. If your cupping is too strong you can loosen the suction by using this pressing method to allow a little air into the cup.

9. Remove any oil with a clean piece of couch roll.

10. Wash the cups after use with Milton's solution.

Apply cupping before Tui na treatment. Once the cups have been removed, work gently to soothe the area and to help to disperse local stagnation, then continue with the rest of your Tui na treatment.

Cupping marks

Cupping will often leave a reddish-purple, circular, bruise-like mark the first time it is applied, unless a weak method is being used or there is no stagnation or pathogen present. It is important that you warn your patient about this and reassure them that the marks will fade after a few days. The color of the mark depends partly on the strength of cupping applied and also on the amount of stagnation present. Usually after cupping has been applied three or four times the marks become gradually less apparent, and eventually, when the stagnation moves or the pathogen clears, there will be no marks at all.

Once I had a patient with a frozen shoulder who had so much stagnation of Qi and Blood that his cup marks were black at first. As treatment progressed, these went from black to purple to red and, eventually one day, there was nothing. The marks in themselves are very useful diagnostically.

The strength of the suction is altered by the size of the flame and the time you leave the flame in the cup. The bigger the flame, the stronger the suction.

There are several cupping methods and the ones that are relevant to Tui na are described below.

Weak cupping

A gentle suction is applied – just enough to hold the cups in place. This is used for patients who are very Deficient, frail or old. This method should not create any redness or bruising to the patient's skin.

Medium cupping

This is the most commonly used form. A moderate suction is applied so you can see that the skin is raised up a little inside the cup. This method is suitable for most patients. It will generally produce some red cupping marks. It can also be applied to the abdomen for digestive problems such as Middle Jiao disharmony.

Strong cupping

This is only applied to patients with strong constitutions and purely Excess conditions and is therefore rarely used. It is applied for only 3–5 minutes. Never apply strong cupping the first time you cup a patient; it can be very draining and will generally produce a lot of red and purple cupping marks.

Empty or walking cupping

This is a very useful method if you have a patient who is both Deficient and has a lot of Qi stagnation. It invigorates the Qi but does not drain it. It is commonly applied to the back along the Bladder channel and Governing Vessel. Several cups, usually between five and 10, are applied one after another in quick succession. Each cup only remains in place for a few seconds before it is removed and replaced at a different site. The cups are kept continually moving on and off the body for about 5 minutes (Fig. 8.2).

Moving or sliding cupping

This is a strong method of cupping and can be painful if the suction applied is too strong. It is generally used for Excess Heat conditions and can create some quite dramatic looking purple red marks. The cups are applied and then slid up and down the area to be treated. It is usually applied to the back (Fig. 8.3).

Therapeutic effects of cupping

- Regulates and invigorates the flow of Qi and Blood
- Moves stagnant Qi and Blood
- Eases pain
- Relaxes the muscles
- Draws out and releases pathogenic Wind, Cold, Damp and Heat

Suggestions for use

- Common colds, coughs and flu
- Chronic bronchitis and asthma
- Muscular pain and tension
- Bi syndrome
- Lower backache
- Frozen shoulder
- Tennis elbow
- Digestive weakness
- Irregular menstruation and dysmenorrhea

Contraindications

Do not apply cupping:
- To areas of skin where there is a skin disease such as psoriasis or eczema or if the skin is burnt
- To the abdomen or lower back during pregnancy
- If the patient is very weak

Note on safety

Remember you are dealing with fire. Take your time and pay attention to what you are doing. Make sure the cotton wool ball is not dripping with surgical spirits – squeeze out any excess before you begin.

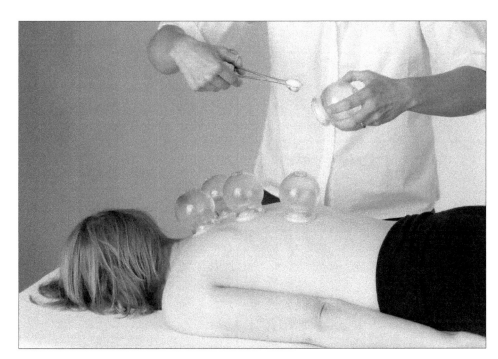

Fig. 8.1 Application of cupping.

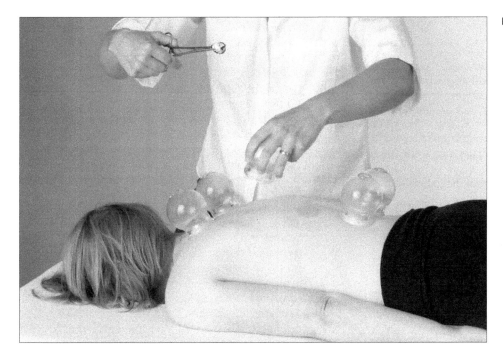

Fig. 8.2 Empty cupping.

Gua sha

Gua sha is a similar therapy to cupping in that it is used to release the Exterior, expel pathogens and move stagnant Qi and Blood. I use it a great deal in my practice and have found it extremely effective in the treatment of migraine and hypertension as well as for a variety of muscular skeletal problems. It is a very flexible and highly effective therapy to use in conjunction with Tui na.

'Gua' means to scrape or scratch and 'sha' is 'a red, elevated, hot skin rash'. The rash or petechia is intention-ally brought to the surface by scraping the patient's skin with a rounded tool. This sounds worse than it actually is; it is in fact painless when done correctly and patients often find it very relieving, as it is so effective for easing pain and stiffness.

Gua sha affects the Exterior of the body, the Wei Qi level and channel sinews. It has been used in many countries as part of folk medicine for treating common ailments such as fever, common colds, aches and pains. Towards the end of the last century, Jingluo gua sha was developed and used by practitioners of Chinese medicine both as a diagnostic method and for the treatment of painful conditions such as Bi syndrome.

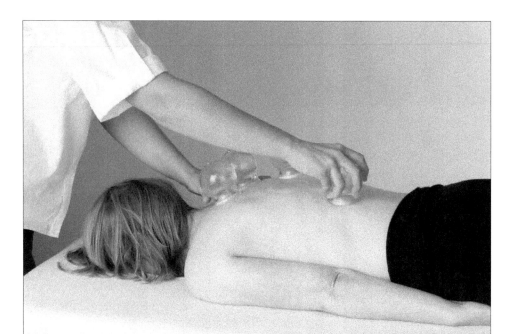

Fig. 8.3 Cupping–sliding.

The 'sha' or rash

Gua sha marks can look quite dramatic. The red or purple rash is a sign that Qi and Blood are obstructed and not circulating properly. As with cupping it is important to warn your patient about the marks and explain the purpose of what you are doing. The sha should fade in 3–4 days unless there is pronounced Blood stasis. Do not apply gua sha again to the treated area until the marks have completely gone.

The color of the sha is a useful diagnostic tool:

- **Very light sha** indicates Blood Deficiency
- **Red sha** indicates a recent invasion of a pathogenic factor
- **Dark red sha** usually indicates Heat
- **Purple or very dark sha** indicates long-standing Blood stasis

How to apply gua sha

Gua sha is applied with a round-edged implement that is blunt and smooth. Originally, metal coins and porcelain Chinese soup spoons were used until specific gua sha tools were made from buffalo horn and jade. Gua sha is applied primarily to the Yang surfaces of the body: the back, neck, shoulders, buttocks and limbs. However, it can also be applied to the chest and abdomen.

How to apply gua sha (Fig. 8.4):

1. Apply red flower, white flower or woodlock oil to the area to be treated. Red flower is particularly good for gua sha, but choose the oil according to the disharmony.
2. Hold your gua sha tool in your dominant hand, keeping an angle of 45 degrees between the tool and the skin.
3. Scrape the area to be treated firmly, gently and smoothly using short, brisk strokes. If you are applying gua sha to the spine or other bony areas use lighter pressure.
4. Work along or across channels from top to bottom and from the midline out.
5. Keep scraping until the sha appears then move on to the next area. If there is no Blood stasis, the petechiae will not form and the skin will only turn pink. If you are working on a large area, for example on the back along the Governing Vessel and Bladder channels, the whole process will take about 15–20 minutes.
6. After you have finished, apply Tui na to soothe the area and to clear and disperse the released stagnation, using techniques like Tui fa, Gun fa and Ca fa.
7. If you want to strengthen Wei Qi, apply gua sha along the Governing Vessel and Bladder channels in long, gentle strokes.
8. Clean your gua sha tool after use with Milton's solution.

Therapeutic effects

- Releases the Exterior and expels pathogenic factors
- Invigorates and moves Qi and Blood
- Breaks up areas of congestion, stagnation and stasis
- Relaxes and releases the channel sinews
- Eases pain
- Descends Yang
- Strengthens the Wei Qi
- Clears Heat
- Regulates the functions of the Stomach and Spleen

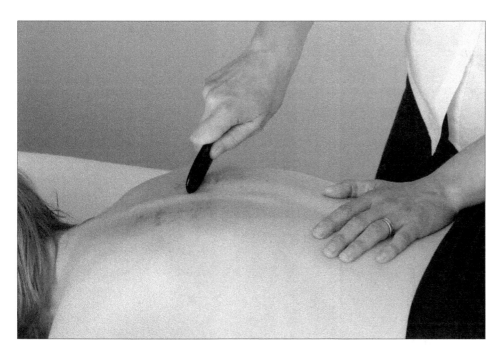

Fig. 8.4 Gua sha on the back.

Moxibustion

Suggestions for use

Gua sha is probably the most effective way of moving stagnation. Use it to treat:

- Any acute or chronic pain, stiffness and immobility
- Sunstroke
- Fever
- Colds and flu
- Bronchitis, asthma and emphysema
- Headaches and migraine
- Hypertension

Use it to prevent:

- Invasions of pathogenic factors
- Stagnation and to improve circulation

Contraindications

Do not apply gua sha:

- To areas of skin where there is a skin disease such as psoriasis or eczema or if the skin is burnt
- Over areas where there are moles, broken skin, cuts and bruises or other blemishes
- To the abdomen or lower back during pregnancy
- If the patient is very weak

Moxibustion

Moxibustion involves burning a dried herb, usually mugwort, either directly onto the skin or indirectly above the skin, to stimulate and warm specific points, channels or areas of the body. Moxa can be bought in a loose form or in pre-rolled sticks. There are several varieties of loose moxa or moxa 'punk' available; some are quite coarse and others very refined. The coarse moxa is good for making large cones to be applied on top of ginger, garlic and salt, and the fine quality, often Japanese moxa, is excellent for point stimulation and tonification.

Moxibustion has been used in China for thousands of years by practitioners of Chinese medicine and plays a very important role in the traditional medical systems of Japan, Korea, Vietnam, Tibet and Mongolia. Tui na and moxibustion date back long before the invention of needles and acupuncture. Chinese medicine practitioners have used these therapies in conjunction for thousands of years.

How to apply moxibustion

There are several ways of applying moxa. The methods commonly used in conjunction with Tui na are:

- Direct moxibustion with cones
- Indirect moxibustion
- With cones over ginger, garlic or salt
- With a moxa stick
- With a moxa box

Direct moxibustion with cones

1. Knead and shape the loose moxa into a cone. The size of the cones will vary according to the purpose of treatment. Cones the size of a grain of rice are used for point stimulation and tonification; larger cones the size of half an olive or bigger are used for heating and increasing Yang.
2. Dip your little finger in water and dab it onto the point to be treated: this will help the cone to stay in place.
3. Place the cone directly onto the skin and light it with an akebane or incense stick (Fig. 8.5).

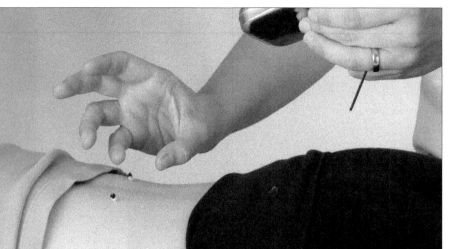

Fig. 8.5 Direct moxa on a point.

4. Ask the patient to tell you when it feels hot. Watch it burn down and be ready to remove it immediately when the patient says 'hot'. If you are using tiny cones this will only take a couple of seconds.

5. To remove the cones, hold a moxa tray in one hand and remove the cone with the other, either with forceps or, as I prefer, by pinching it off between your thumb and little finger (in other words, not your pulse-taking fingers). Repeat this process as many times as required. Generally three cones are enough for point stimulation and general tonification.

6. Apply Tui na point-stimulating techniques such as Yi zhi chan tui fa, Rou fa or Yin style point holding after moxibustion.

This method is commonly used in the treatment of chronic diseases of a Deficient and Cold nature. If the patient has an Excess Cold pathology you can blow on the cones as they burn, to help disperse the Cold.

Indirect moxibustion with cones

Medium to large cones are placed on a slice of ginger, garlic or a mound of salt.

Moxa on ginger

1. Cut a thin slice of fresh ginger about 0.2–0.3 cm thick and place it on the selected point.
2. Put a moxa cone onto the ginger slice.
3. Light the moxa and let it burn down until the patient feels it is too hot. If the patient is very cold, it can take a few cones before they feel the heat. On average 3–5 cones are usually enough, but it can take as many as 10. The skin will become flushed and wet as an indication that enough treatment has

been given. This method is frequently used for Yang Xu, Cold in the Middle or Lower Jiao and Wind-Damp-Cold Bi syndrome. (Fig. 8.6)

Moxa on garlic

1. Cut a slice of garlic about 0.1–0.2 cm thick.
2. Put the garlic slice onto the selected point with a moxa cone on top.
3. Light the cone and burn as above. Renew the slice of garlic each time three moxa cones are burnt out. This method is very effective for Damp conditions and relieving swelling.

Moxa on salt

1. Fill the navel with salt.
2. Place a large moxa cone on top of the salt, light it and burn down as above.
3. Ask the patient to tell you when they feel the heat inside their abdomen, not just on the surface. Generally 3–9 cones are applied. If the salt becomes very encrusted, remove a little and replace it with some fresh salt.
4. Leave the warm salt in the navel until the end of the treatment.
5. To remove the salt, put a piece of couch roll over your patient's navel and ask them to turn onto one side and tip the salt into the couch roll.

This method is very effective for warming and strengthening Yang, for warming the Uterus and for strengthening the Spleen. I have found it very useful for supporting the Shen and helping patients to come back into their own center. This is the method used to restore Yang in acute cases of Yang collapse.

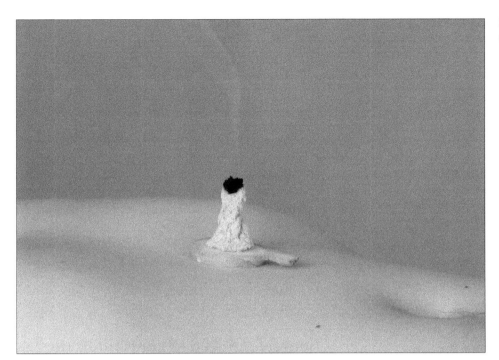

Fig. 8.6 Indirect moxa on ginger.

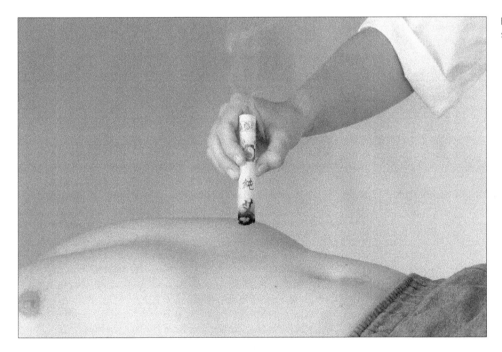

Fig. 8.7 Indirect moxa with a stick.

Indirect moxibustion with moxa sticks

Moxibustion with a moxa stick (Fig. 8.7) is easy to apply; patients generally like it and it has a very good therapeutic effect.

Light the end of the moxa stick and hold it about 3 cm above the selected point. Hold the stick securely but not too tightly, it is important to keep relaxed and allow your Qi to flow through your arm and hand as you would if you were applying Tui na. You can apply it in four different ways:

1. Still point warming

Hold the stick above the point for 5–15 minutes until the skin around the point becomes flushed. It should feel pleasantly warming and comfortable.

2. Sparrow-pecking

Hold the stick above the point and then peck up and down like a sparrow pecking at seeds. This can be applied rapidly or more slowly and deliberately. Think of throwing the moxa smoke and Qi into the point. It is generally applied for between 3–5 minutes. Thinking of the application of Ji dian fa will help you to perfect this method.

3. Circling

Hold the moxa stick above the point or area to be treated and circle the stick in a clockwise direction for between 5–20 minutes. Think of the application of Mo fa.

4. Channel warming

Hold the stick over the channel and move it gradually and smoothly along the section to be treated, for example, for tennis elbow from LI11 to LI1. Apply this for 5–10 minutes or until the area becomes hot to touch. Thinking of the application of Tui fa will help you to perfect this method.

Moxibustion using a moxa box

1. Either cut a moxa stick into small pieces about 1–3 cm in length, or make several large cones out of loose moxa.
2. Light one end of the small moxa stick pieces and put them into the moxa box. Or if you are using cones, put them in the box first and then light them with an akebane stick.
3. Put the moxa box onto the lower back or abdomen.

The moxa is burnt over a wire mesh inside the box; this allows the warming effect of the moxa to gradually penetrate a wide area. This method is commonly used to treat back pain from Kidney-Yang Deficiency and diarrhea from Kidney- and Spleen-Yang Deficiency.

Therapeutic effects

Moxa is Yang, hot, strong and supportive in nature. It can be applied to:

- Stimulate the actions of the points and gently tonify and nourish Qi and Blood
- Strengthen and warm Yang
- Rescue Yang
- Raise Qi
- Activate the circulation of Qi and Blood
- Rectify and regulate the flow of Qi and Blood
- Move stagnation and clear obstructions
- Warm the channels
- Dissipate Cold
- Resolve Damp
- Relax the muscles
- Ease pain and swelling
- Strengthen Wei Qi

Suggestions for use

The application of moxa is extremely wide ranging. Some common uses:

- Wind-Damp-Cold Bi syndrome
- Channel sinew problems due to stagnation
- Lower backache due to Yang Xu or Qi and Blood stagnation
- Infertility due to Kidney-Yang Xu and a Cold Uterus
- Dysmenorrhea
- Diarrhea
- Hemorrhoids and other prolapses
- Poor digestion
- Stroke sequelae
- Muscular atrophy
- Tiredness
- Qi and Blood Deficiency
- Turning breech babies

General points and contraindications

- Moxibustion is generally applied in the following order:
  - To the upper part of the body first and then the lower part
  - The back first, then the abdomen
  - The head first and then the limbs
  - The Yang channels, then the Yin channels.
- Never use moxa on an individual with signs of Full Heat, such as a bright-red tongue, rapid pulse, thirst and fever.
- If a patient has Yin Xu, be cautious with your application of moxa. The application of very heating methods such as a moxa box is contraindicated. However, the application of a minimum of direct rice grain cones to stimulate and tonify points is, in my experience, quite acceptable and often beneficial. In fact, patients with Empty Heat symptoms and cold feet, such as women with menopausal hot flushes, respond very well to the application of moxa to points on their feet such as Taichong Liv3.
- Occasionally the skin may blister after the application of direct moxa. If this happens, generally the blisters are small and heal by themselves.
- Do not use moxa if the patient has hypertension or other Yang rising symptoms, unless their feet are cold, then apply moxa only to their feet. In these circumstances, you are using heat to draw heat down.

CHAPTER **9**

External herbs

Andrew Croysdale

Introduction

All cultures have a history of using herbs externally. Many people have used dock leaves for a stinging nettle sting as a child. Much of this knowledge has been lost in the West but China has preserved its knowledge, which has been continuously developed over the centuries. That, coupled with its vast array of flora and fauna, makes this an extremely interesting subject to learn. The use of external herbs, various oils, tinctures and washes form an important part of the Tui na therapist's practice, aiding and increasing the effectiveness of treatments and enabling the patient to self-treat by applying various products supplied by the practitioner. There are many pre-made products on the market for use in Tui na, but actually producing your own brings something special to the healing process. It is also a very pleasurable thing to do. The formulas that are presented here have been passed onto me by various teachers over the years and I am extremely happy to pass on some of these tried and tested recipes.

Contraindications

The following contraindications apply to all of the herbal formulas in this chapter. Traditionally, herbal products may be applied during pregnancy but not over the abdomen. Virtually all external herbs, apart from ginger compress, have blood-moving properties; the early stages of a fetus are perceived in Chinese medicine as a clot, and therefore blood-moving herbs are not used on the abdomen. I never use external herbs during pregnancy because the herbs absorb into the bloodstream of the mother through the skin and via the blood into the baby.

Do not apply any herbs where the skin is broken, there is eczema or psoriasis, or there are any boils or spots present. Always ask the patient if they have sensitive skin or any particular allergies. If in doubt, apply a very small amount of the herb you are going to use to see if there is any reaction.

Contusions or bumps on the head can be effectively treated with Tui na and external herbs but the patient must first go to the hospital to be X-rayed and checked for concussion.

Oils

Sesame oil toasted

This is traditionally used to moisten the skin during massage, and is widely available at health food stores. It is generally applied to the back and abdomen, with techniques such as Ca fa *scrubbing* and Mo fa *sliding*.

Traditional Chinese medicine (TCM) actions:
Moistens dry skin, strengthens the Spleen and nourishes Blood.
Safe to use during pregnancy

Turpentine oil

This is the natural turpentine collected from pine trees, not the synthetic kind used as a solvent for paints. It may be obtained from builders' merchants but you must specify that it is the pure natural form you require. It is applied using a variety of techniques to the skin at the joint area, or where there are sore or injured muscles and rheumatic pains. When applying the oil with the Ca fa *scrubbing* technique, stop when you begin to feel friction, so as not to burn the skin.

TCM actions:
Clears and expels Wind, reduces Dampness and swelling, relaxes muscles and tendons and invigorates Blood flow.
Contraindicated during pregnancy

White flower oil

This is a pre-made patent formula and can be bought from any Chinese supermarket or herbal supplier. It can be applied to all areas, including the face, and is mainly used on acupuncture points with gentle massage.

Ingredients:
Menthol, camphor, borneal, lavender oil, methyl salicylate, eucalyptus oil and liquid paraffin.

TCM actions:
Invigorates the body and mind, relaxes muscles and tendons, clears the sinuses, stops bleeding and stops aches and pains.

Treats:
Headache, cold and flu, nausea, muscular aches and pain, burns and cuts, stomach and abdominal pains.
Contraindicated during pregnancy

Red flower oil

This is a pre-made preparation which can be purchased at any Chinese herbalist, and is widely available in Chinese supermarkets or from oriental herbal suppliers.

Ingredients:
Liquid paraffin, cassia oil, cinnamon leaf oil, turpentine, cinnamic aldehyde, wintergreen oil and dragon's blood resin.

How to use:
Pour a few drops into your hand. Apply to the affected area. Massage in using either the Mo fa *round rubbing* or Ca fa *scrubbing* technique on broader areas like the lower back for 4–8 minutes.

TCM actions:
Relieves pain, relaxes muscles and tendons, invigorates Blood flow and stops bleeding.

Treats:
Lower backache, muscular pain, arthritis, Wind-Cold Bi syndrome, insect and mosquito bites, minor cuts and burns.
Contraindicated during pregnancy

Woodlock oil

This pre-prepared formula sometimes has slightly different ingredients, depending on the manufacturer, but all will have the same action. It can be purchased from the usual sources.

Ingredients:
Methyl salicylate, menthol, turpentine oil and camphor. Some also have the addition of clove oil.

How to use:
Place a few drops into the palm and rub lightly into the affected area. Over-rubbing can cause skin burn and over-application may result in palpitations, especially if clove oil is present.

TCM actions:
Resolves Blood stasis, invigorates Blood flow, relaxes sinews and tendons, warms and disperses Cold and relieves pain.

Treats:
Bruising, unopened trauma, muscular aches and pains and sprains.
Contraindicated during pregnancy

Juices

Juices of vegetables and roots are a useful asset in a Tui na treatment. They are generally always to hand in the kitchen or local shop. They are very simple to prepare and use, inexpensive and highly effective at enhancing a treatment. All juices should be applied with light Mo fa.

Preparation:
To prepare the vegetable or root, first wash and peel it if required, and then grate, pound or liquidize it. Place in a piece of linen cloth, and then twist and squeeze out the juice into a dish. Any left-over juice can be stored in the fridge for a few days.

Spring onion

TCM actions:
Its properties are pungent and warm. It induces perspiration, releases the Exterior, invigorates energy and refreshes the spirit.

Treats:
Applied over the abdomen area, it releases the Exterior and will clear common colds. Applied to Fengchi GB20 and Dazhui Du14 with a needling technique, it will clear headache and stuffy nose. It will also treat abdominal pain and dysuria.
Safe to use during pregnancy

Ginger

Its properties are pungent and slightly warm. It also releases the Exterior, clears Cold, warms the Middle Burner and stops nausea.

Treats:
When rubbed into the neck and shoulders using the points GB20 and Du14 and BL12, it treats stiffness of the neck, headache and the common cold. If rubbed over the chest it will cure cough with retention of phlegm. When applied on the Ren Mai meridian from Ren10 to Ren13 and to the abdominal area it will cure abdominal pain, vomiting, diarrhea and abdominal bloating.
Safe to use during pregnancy

Note on green ginger

Green ginger can be used to treat a Wind-Cold invasion of the neck and shoulders. Cut a thick slice of green ginger root, about 5 cm in diameter, and peel off the skin. This is then used to perform gua sha over the affected areas. Scrape briskly down from GB20 to GB21. Repeat the process until the sha comes to the surface. Apply also down the Bladder meridian. The ginger juice acts as its own lubricant, warming and dispersing the Wind-Cold. I have had great success with this method and use it regularly. It is always good in an emergency.

The other use of a green ginger slice is to treat damaged tendons and ligaments. Perform gua sha over the tendons and ligaments for up to 5 minutes. The tendons will be warmed, lubricated and relaxed. Red areas will appear over the tendons or ligaments. This will indicate where the main damage is and further Tui na manipulation may be applied.

Garlic

Its properties are pungent and warm. It clears stagnant Qi, warms the Middle Burner, strengthens the Stomach energy, reduces swelling and clears athlete's foot and fungal disorders. When applied to Ren17 and BL3 it treats common cold and cough. Two slices of garlic can be applied to Yongquan KD1 with a sticking plaster to clear colds and flu.

Safe to use during pregnancy

Peppermint

Its properties are pungent and cool. It clears Wind and cools Heat. It invigorates energy, and releases the Exterior. When applied to the temples and forehead it will treat Wind-Heat headache and stuffy nose. Around the throat region, it will soothe a sore throat.

Safe to use during pregnancy

Herbal compresses

Herbal compresses are the application of a folded flannel soaked in hot water in which herbs have been steeped. This is then covered with a towel allowing the herbs and heat to be slowly released into the desired area. This is generally used for acute Wind-Cold invasions, swelling, lower back pain and to release the Exterior. It is an extremely easy process to perform and brings rapid relief. It is great in an emergency as very simple herbs can be used, such as ginger, cinnamon, mugwort and spring onion.

Equipment

- Stove or cooker for boiling water and herbs – in the clinic, a flat-based camping stove is preferable, as safety is important when you have hot water boiling close to a patient
- Four to five toweling flannels for the compress
- A pair of tongs
- A lidded, airtight container to store the hot herbal liquid and keep it as hot as possible
- Two to three large towels per patient
- The herbs you need for your compress
- A small table or surface between yourself and the patient; this will ensure that any splashes or spillages are well away from you and your patient

Preparation

1. Take four cups of water and bring to the boil.
2. If herbs are dry, simmer for 20 minutes to extract the goodness of the herbs.
3. If herbs are fresh, take the water off the boil and add the freshly extracted herbal juice of the herbs you are using. This allows the vitality of the herb to be preserved.
4. Strain the hot liquid into a plastic lidded container. This will keep it hot longer. The straining is only essential with the hard herbs, as these will feel uncomfortable on the skin.
5. Place one flannel in the liquid, replace the lid and wait 30–40 seconds.
6. Use the tongs to remove the flannel by a corner of the flannel.
7. Allow excess water to drain. If it is too hot, take the other corner and open out the flannel, wave it back and forth three or four times and release one corner. With the other hand, grip the flannel lightly at the top and run your hand down its length quickly. This will remove excess hot liquid that could splash on your patient. Your hand will also tell you if it is too hot to put on the patient. If it burns, open it out and wave back and forth another three or four times. Fold the flannel into three along one length. Immediately place over the selected area on the patient's bare skin and cover with a towel. Place another flannel in the container and close the lid. This will be hot and ready for when your first flannel cools.

Sometimes two or three areas need to be compressed at the same time, most typically the nape of the neck, the neck and shoulders, or neck and lower back or both knees and abdomen.

The flannels will cool quite quickly. Ask the patient how hot it is. When it cools initially, pat over the towel several times to release the heat and herbs inside. When it begins to cool, have the second flannel squeezed of excess liquid and folded, ready. Lift the towel, remove the cold flannel and replace it with the hot one. Cover with the towel, place the cold flannel in the hot liquid and replace the lid.

When two or more areas are to be compressed, place two to three flannels in the pot.

Keep the process going until the liquid begins to become too cool to be used; this should be at least after three to four applications per area. Then remove all flannels and dry the area with a towel. Relevant points can be stimulated and other areas worked on while the compress is in place.

Ginger juice compress

Grate a large handful of ginger. Once the water is boiled, take it off the heat and squeeze the juice into the pan. Transfer this to your container.

TCM actions:
It will release the Exterior at the early stages of the Wind-Cold invasion.

Treats:
It will release and relieve a stiff neck, lower backache and any areas affected by Wind and Cold. It is used abdominally to relieve period pains and against nausea. If no green ginger is available, dry ginger can be used but must be placed in the water and boiled for 10 minutes. Cinnamon powder can be added for extra warmth at the boiling stage.
Safe to use during pregnancy

Moxa compress (mugwort)

It can be used dried or fresh. Add 9 g of moxa to boiling water, 3 minutes for fresh, 5 minutes for dry. Remove and strain into your container.

TCM actions:
Moves Qi and Blood.

Treats:
This is used to treat torticollis and acute Wind-Cold invasion of the neck and other parts of the body. In severe cases the whole compress process might be repeated again.
Contraindicated during pregnancy

Herbal decoction/hot compress for lumbar problems

Ingredients:
Dang gui **30 g** *Radix angelicaesinensis*
Chen xiang **30 g** *Aquilaria agallocha Roxb*
Fang ji **30 g** *Stephaniae radix*
Kuan jing teng **30 g** *Ramulus tinospora sinensis*
Gui zhi **30 g** *Cinnamomi cassiae ramulus*
Lu lu tong **30 g** *Liquidambaris fructus*
Ji xue teng **30 g** *Spatholobi caulis et radix*
You song jie **30 g** *Lignum pini nodi*
Shen jin cao **30 g** *Herba Lycopodii*
Wei ling xian **30 g** *Clematidis radix*
Gan jiang **30 g** *Zingiberis rhizoma*
Sang zhi **30 g** *Mori ramulus*

Preparation:
Place 30 g of each herb in water and soak for 30 minutes. Bring to the boil. Once boiling, simmer for 20–30 minutes, then use over the affected part of the lumbar area. The decoction can be used for 1 week, or if not being used, it can be frozen, as with other herbal compresses.
Contraindicated during pregnancy

Compress for obstruction of Excess Cold in the Uterus

Ingredients:
Jiang huang **10 g** *Rhizoma curcumae longa*
Rou gui **6 g** *Cortex cinnamomi*
Gan jiang **10 g** *Zingiberis rhizoma*
Fu tzu **6–10 g** *Radix aconiti lateralis*

TCM actions:
Moves Blood stasis and clears Cold. Warms and invigorates the Uterus.

Treats:
Period pains and abdominal pains.
Contraindicated during pregnancy

Gaos (*ointments*)

Ointments are extremely important for the Tui na practitioner. Not only do they lubricate the manipulation, they hold the herbs within the ointment on the skin for longer, allowing greater absorption of the active ingredients. Typically, ointments are applied at the end of a Tui na treatment. They also have the added advantage that once you have diagnosed the patient's problem you can send them away with some of the ointment for regular application, further enhancing the treatment's effectiveness until you see the patient again. All ointments comprise a base medium. It can be sesame oil, Vaseline, beeswax or some form of animal fat. Herbal extracts are added to the base; the base facilitates long-term storage and also acts as the lubricating medium.

Dong qing gao

This is probably one of the most famous Tui na balms used today. Unfortunately, it is not readily available on the market as with its counterparts, Tiger balm and essential balm. This means the active ingredients have to be bought and made at home.

Ingredients:
Menthol crystals **20 g**
Methyl salicylate **20 g**
Vaseline **100 g**

Preparation:
Grind the menthol crystals into a fine powder. Melt the Vaseline over a low heat. Once melted add the menthol crystals and methyl salicylate (wintergreen). It is important to keep the temperature very low because at this stage it is flammable. Stir, and once the crystals have dissolved, remove from the heat. Allow to cool before placing into brown glass jars with a tight top. This is because wintergreen will dissolve certain plastics, including the vinyl on your couch, so care must be taken with its use. Always wash your hands after use. The last thing you want to do is scratch your eye with the ointment still on your fingers.

How to use:
Take a small amount of the ointment and rub it between the palms. It is generally applied with the Ca fa *scrubbing* technique over large areas like the lumbar region, up and down the spine or the backs of the thighs until heat is generated. For smaller areas it can be applied by using sword finger Ca fa.

TCM actions:
Warms and relaxes the muscles, invigorates Qi and promotes Blood flow. Disperses stagnant energy.

Treats:
Use for any aches or pains, sciatica, strained muscles, insect bites and lower backache. It can be placed on acupuncture points to keep them active longer.
Contraindicated during pregnancy

Golden glowing ointment

Ingredients:
Menthol crystals **20 g**
Camphor crystals **20 g**
Eucalyptus oil **20 g**
Vaseline **100 g**
Beeswax **40 g**

Preparation:
Preparation is as for dong qing gao.

How to use:
As for dong qing gao. It is not as warming as dong qing gao.

TCM actions:
Disperses Damp and resolves swelling, clears Blood stasis, relieves pain, and relaxes muscles and tendons.

Treats:
Sprained ankles, muscular pain, swollen knees, insect bites, stomach ache, abdominal pains and nausea.

Contraindicated during pregnancy

Ointment for asthma with heat

Ingredients:
Ban bian lian **10 g** *Herba lobelia chinensis*
Kuan dong hua **10 g** *Tussilaginis farfarae*
Horehound **10 g** *Marrubium vulgare*
Mullein **10 g** *Verbascum thapsus*
Benzoin **6 g** (ground fine)
Lavender oil **7 drops**
Eucalyptus oil **7 drops**
Beeswax **100 g**
Sesame oil **1 liter**

Preparation:
Take a 1-liter bottle of sesame oil. Fry the herbs at a low heat slowly until dark brown but not burnt. Strain the mixture, then add the beeswax or equivalent base while the mixture is still warm, adding also the benzoin, lavender oil and eucalyptus oil. Stir until they all dissolve. Pour the mixture into a brown glass jar.

TCM actions:
Descends Qi, clears Heat and resolves Phlegm.

Treats:
For asthma with Heat, rub onto the chest area.
Note: This is one of my teacher's formulas and I have not yet had the need or opportunity to prepare it or use it. It is certainly contraindicated for use during pregnancy or in a person with Lung-Heat due to Yin Deficiency. I have added it here so some benefit can be obtained from the formula.
Contraindicated during pregnancy

Essential balm

This is a famous balm that you can buy over the counter and it is even available in Western chemists and shops. The ingredients are combined in a base and the balm comes in a small red tin. It is a must for any traveler.

Ingredients:
Menthol **14%**
Camphor **14%**
Peppermint oil **8%**
Eucalyptus oil **8%**
Clove oil **4%**

How to use:
Massage a small amount into the affected area using a light circular motion.

TCM actions:
Eases pains and aches, warms muscles and relaxes tendons, clears the sinus and relieves insect and mosquito bites.

Treats:
Headache and migraine, muscle pain, blocked sinuses, hayfever, insect bites and sprains.
Contraindicated during pregnancy

Tinctures

Traditionally, tinctures are herbal formulas that have been soaked in either wine or spirit for a certain length of time until the active ingredients within the herbs permeate the liquid. This is then strained, bottled and stored for future use. They keep indefinitely and are extremely easy to apply. This category also comprises the Dit Da Jiao which are, traditionally, formulas used by martial artists of different styles to treat various traumatic injuries. Each school would have developed several types for different purposes and they were a jealously guarded secret.

Release the Exterior rub for common cold

Ingredients:
A large handful of chopped fresh spring onions
A large handful of chopped fresh ginger
Chinese white spirit **0.5 liter** (vodka or surgical spirit can be used as an alternative)

Preparation:
Add the onions and ginger to the bottle of spirit. Let it stand for one moon cycle in a dark warm place. Strain and squeeze the residue and the rub is ready to use. This will store indefinitely.

How to use:
This is rubbed over the whole of the abdomen and the sides using Mo fa *round rubbing* technique, until the liquid is absorbed. I prefer to repeat this process three times after stimulating points to release the Exterior, then requesting that the patient goes home to bed with extra covers to sweat out the pathogens. If the patient comes early in the morning, give them some in a small container and direct them to use it before they go to bed. After one application, sheets on the bed must be changed. This is extremely

effective on young children and can be used during pregnancy.

TCM actions:
Releases the Exterior, opens the pores, induces sweating and warms the Middle and Lower Jiao.

Treats:
Common cold and flu.
Safe to use during pregnancy

Disperse Wind and scatter Cold (acute invasion)

Ingredients:
Dang gui **12 g** *Radix angelicae sinensis*
Du huo **12 g** *Radix angelicae pubescentis*
Hua jiao **12 g** *Fructus sophorae*
Fang feng **12 g** *Radix ledebouriellae*
Mo yao **12 g** *Myrrhae*
Jing jie **9 g** *Herba schizonepetae*
Ma huang **3 g** *Herba ephedrae* (or replace with Gui zhi 9 g)
Hong hua **9 g** *Flos carthami*
Qiang huo **12 g** *Rhizoma seu radix notopterygii*
Shen jin cao **12 g** *Herba Lycopodii*
Hai feng teng **12 g** *Caulis piperis*
Sang zhi **12 g** *Ramulus mori albae* (white mulberry twig)
Alcohol 60%
Chinese spirit **1.5 liters** (alternatively vodka or surgical spirit)

Preparation:
Add all the ingredients to the alcohol and allow to soak for 3 months. Strain off the quantities you need for use and leave the rest of the herbs in the spirit to build up more potency.

How to use:
Rub into the affected area using Mo fa or Ca fa.

TCM actions:
Disperses Wind, scatters Cold, unblocks channels, invigorates Blood, unblocks the sinuses and stops pain.

Treats:
Acute Wind-Cold-Damp Bi syndrome in which Wind and Cold are the major pathogenic factors, e.g. rheumatism, swelling of the knees and ankles and muscular traumas of the legs and waist. Torticollis and sciatica. Aches and sprains.
Contraindicated during pregnancy

Scatter Cold, disperse Blood stasis and clear Damp

Ingredients:
Dang gui **9 g** *Radix angelicae sinensis*
Jiang huang **9 g** *Rhizoma curcumae longae*
Hong hua **12 g** *Flos carthami*
Chuan niu xi **12 g** *Radix cyathulae officinalis*
Rou gui **12 g** *Cortex cinnamomi*
Mo yao **12 g** *Myrrhae*
Zhi shi **12 g** *Fructus aurantii immaturus*
Huo xiang **12 g** *Agastaches seu pogostemi herba*

Preparation:
Place herbs in the bottle and soak for 3 months. Strain off the amount needed.

How to use:
Apply with light Mo fa until herbs are absorbed.

TCM actions:
Warms and scatters Cold, disperses stasis, transforms swelling and stops pain.

Treats:
Wind-Cold-Damp Bi syndrome, bruising with swelling, damaged tendons and ligaments, injuries to the lower back, waist, legs, ankles and upper limbs. Excellent for sprained ankles.
Contraindicated during pregnancy

Abdominal problems

Ingredients:
Rou gui **9 g** *Cortex cinnamomi*
Bai zhi **6 g** *Radix angelicae dahuricae*
Wu zhu yu **9 g** *Fructus evodiae*
Gao liang jiang **9 g** *Rhizoma alpiniae officinarum*
Qing pi **9 g** *Pericarpium citri reticulatae viride*
Menthol crystals **3 g**
Jiang huang **6 g** *Rhizoma curcumae longae*
Xi xin **6 g** *Herba asari*

Preparation:
Place herbs in the bottle and soak for 3 months. Strain off the amount needed.

How to use:
Apply with light Mo fa until herbs are absorbed.

TCM actions:
Moves Qi and Blood.

Treats:
Any abdominal problems involving stagnation, pain and distension; especially good at treating abdominal distension and any abdominal pains when applied to Shenque Ren8, including premenstrual pain, distension and bloating.
Contraindicated during pregnancy

Herbal plasters

Several herbal plasters are available on the market. These are applied to the skin over an injured area, keeping the herbal preparation active for much longer. Each plaster can be used for up to 24 hours or until they come off naturally. Patients can be given several plasters and can apply them themselves between treatments to increase the effectiveness. Herbal plasters can also be made and used by the practitioner. They will also store for a long time.

Plaster for asthma

Ingredients:
Bai jie zi **15 g** *Semen sinapsis albae*
Xi xin **15 g** *Herba asari*
Gan sui **15 g** *Radix euphorbiae kansui*
Yan hu suo **15 g** *Rhizoma corydalis*

Ding xiang **30 g** *Flos caryophylli*
Rou gui **15 g** *Cortex cinnamomi*

Either buy these in powdered form or grind them as fine as possible. Then mix them with fresh ginger juice to the consistency of a thick paste. This can be stored in an airtight container until needed.

How to use:
Make into flat pills about a centimeter in diameter. These are then applied to BL12, BL13 and BL43 and kept in place with a sticking plaster. This is done once a month for 3 months of the summer and for three summers in succession and the asthma should be resolved.

Contraindicated during pregnancy

Red dragon plaster

This is a very useful formula for very long-term repetitive strain problems such as tennis elbow and plantar fasciitis where the tissue has become severely inflamed and stagnant and does not seem to be clearing with manipulation and other external applications.

Part 1 ingredients:
Dang gui **10 g** *Radix angelicae sinensis*
Pu gong ying **20 g** *Herba taraxaci*
Pearl barley **25 g**
Hong hua **6 g** *Flos carthami*

Part 2 ingredients:
Ground iron pyrites **9 g**
Mo yao **20 g** *Myrrhae*
Xue jie **20 g** *Sanguis draconis*
Ding xian **25 g** *Flos caryophylli*
Sesame oil **2 tablespoons**
Beeswax **3 ounces**
Clove oil **20 drops**
Vaseline **50 g**

Preparation:
Place the part 1 ingredients in a pan, add a pint of water, bring to the boil and simmer slowly. Reduce down to half a cup of liquid. Strain and squeeze the residue as much as possible. Return this liquid to the pan and then add the part 2 ingredients. Stir continuously on a low heat until the beeswax and Vaseline have melted and all the ingredients have formed a thick paste. Place the mixture into a brown glass jar ready for use.

How to use:
Apply a thick coating over the area to be treated. Cover it with a small piece of cling film; this will keep the herbs as moist as possible for longer. Stick the edges of the cling film down with micropore tape and bandage. It should be repeated as often as possible until symptoms subside. It can also be given to the patient to use in between treatments.

TCM actions:
Reduces inflammation, resolves Blood stasis, relaxes the sinews and tendons and clears stagnation.

Treats:
Chronic repetitive strain injuries such as tennis elbow, golfer's elbow, plantar fasciitis.

Contraindicated during pregnancy

SECTION THREE

Tui na treatment – general principles for creating and planning treatments

推拿

CHAPTER **10**

Introduction to Section Three

This section of the book focuses on how to apply Tui na in the treatment of disease. One of the big challenges for Tui na practitioners is making choices: choices about which techniques to apply and how to apply them, choices about which channels, points and parts of the body to work on, in which order and for how long.

I believe it is essential to teach students how to create their own Tui na treatments and develop their own style of practice rather than just following prescribed treatment recipes. If you can apply your knowledge of Chinese medicine, channels and points together with your knowledge of the therapeutic actions of the Tui na techniques and the various approaches to their application, then you will be able to plan a Tui na treatment for any ailment that you are likely to see in practice.

In this section you will find the general principles of Tui na treatment, which can be followed and applied in the treatment of any ailment. The aim is to provide an underlying structure that will help you to create and plan your own Tui na treatments. You will also find aspects of treatment such as working with breath and visualization, nourishing Deficiency and clearing Excess and combining acupuncture and Tui na.

I look at a variety of common complaints and conditions to help illustrate how to formulate and apply Tui na treatments. Each category, for example muscular skeletal ailments, focuses on the key aspects of treatment and provides guidance, tips and suggestions for how you might approach the treatment of common patterns of disharmony. I give suggestions for techniques to consider applying and draw your attention to any important points to bear in mind. Finally, to illustrate how this can work in practice, I have included many examples of Tui na treatments from my own practice (and a couple that have been kindly provided by my colleagues).

Creating a Tui na treatment

During the initial stages of Tui na training there is a lot to learn. Your attention is taken up with learning Chinese medicine theory, channels and points, anatomy and physiology and how to apply the Tui na techniques. You are developing your own strength, flexibility and coordination, and cultivating Qi and learning how to direct it. There comes a point, usually when the techniques are starting to flow quite well, when you begin to think about applying your knowledge and skills to treat disease in real patients. At this point you are likely to have lots of questions about Tui na treatment, such as:

'If the patient has backache, where should I start the treatment?'

'My mother has a frozen shoulder on the right – shall I work on both shoulders?'

'When should I use gua sha?'

Creating Tui na treatments is a challenging and creative process. There are many choices and decisions to be made. Initially, you gather information from your patient through questioning, palpation and observation; then you make a diagnosis. Based on your diagnosis, you decide on a treatment principle and plan, which creates a clear intention and focus for your treatment. The next challenge is to choose the points, channels and areas of the body to treat and which techniques to apply. You also need to remain open to discovering what your hands and heart might discover as you work with your patients.

In Tui na, as with acupuncture, there is no one 'right' way. There are many approaches to diagnosis and treatment. I believe that any approach can work if the practitioner resonates with it, has made his or her own sense of it and is both challenged and captivated by it. Some students, particularly those who have been working with various forms of energy work, healing and Qigong are naturally intuitive and want to start work on the patient immediately so they can follow their hands and intuition and make their diagnosis as they go. Others, often those who are already acupuncturists, prefer to work things out on paper before they start treatment; they relish the process of 'working it all out', and enjoy working methodically to their plan.

I believe in encouraging students to develop their own style and natural abilities, but good Tui na practitioners need to strike a balance between structure and flexibility, maintaining clarity of intention while keeping an open mind. You need to be able to plan a treatment but also able to improvise if your hands and heart make new discoveries as you work on your patient's body and with their Qi.

In my experience of teaching Tui na I have found that students need a simple framework that helps them to think through how to create a Tui na treatment. Having a basic structure to work with prevents the student and newly qualified practitioner from feeling overwhelmed, confused and lost in the labyrinth of treatment possibilities. It is important in these early stages of clinical practice to be clear about what you are trying to do before you start the treatment, so that once you begin to treat, you can relax enough to be able to focus on other aspects of treatment such as directing your intention and Qi through the techniques to the desired level.

Planning treatment

To help you to focus your thoughts and work out your treatments, use the case format provided in this chapter (see Fig. 10.1) and work with the treatment tips and general principles of treatment.

If you are a professional acupuncturist, shiatsu practitioner or practitioner of another system of bodywork studying Tui na, use your patients' cases and work out what you would do if you were treating them with Tui na. If you are a Tui na student, I suggest that before you begin your student clinical practice, you start to work out as many cases as possible and practice creating Tui na treatments. Use the cases in this book, use cases from other books, for example Giovanni Maciocia's books, and use your friends and family members. The more practice you get, the better.

General principles of treatment

The general principles listed below have developed through the clinical experiences of Tui na doctors and practitioners over Tui na's long history and have proved to increase the curative effects of treatment.

I recommend that during your time in the student clinic and in the early days of developing your professional Tui na practice, you work with these principles and discover for yourself their therapeutic value. For those of you with more experience, it is always useful to return to the basics and refresh your knowledge and practice of Tui na.

Follow the three stages of treatment

A balanced treatment moves through three stages: superficial, deep and back to superficial. These stages or levels of treatment are referred to as adaptive, analgesic and dissipative.

Adaptive stage

Start treatment at the Wei Qi level with relatively superficial techniques applied gently and steadily. The adaptive stage is all about the patient and the practitioner adapting to one another. Introduce the patient to treatment gradually so they can begin to relax and allow the energetic connection between you to occur. It is important to honor the power of that initial touch and contact with the patient's Qi.

The adaptive stage is an opportunity to remember to relax, soften, regulate your breath and direct your Qi through your heart into your hands with your treatment intention in mind. Techniques like Tui fa and Rou fa make ideal adaptive techniques to start treatment with.

Analgesic stage

From the adaptive stage, begin to move gradually deeper, becoming more penetrating in both your physical application of the techniques and your directed focus of intention and Qi. This is the core of the treatment where you can affect the Ying Qi, Yuan Qi and Blood levels. As the rhythmic waves of the techniques begin to penetrate, the patient becomes more relaxed and can drift down into a place somewhere between wakefulness and sleep. This allows you to work deeply into points, release muscles, tendons and ligaments, stimulate Qi and Blood and dredge channels.

At this stage of treatment, patients may feel strong Qi sensations or what is commonly described by Tui na patients as 'good pain'. The treatment given at this level helps to relieve pain, which is why I assume it was termed the analgesic stage. Gun fa's versatility makes it an excellent technique to apply as a smooth link between the adaptive and analgesic stages. Strong techniques like elbow Ya fa and Tan bo fa should be applied in the middle of the analgesic stage.

Dissipative stage

The final stage is about coming back up to the surface to the Wei Qi level, breaking up and dissipating any stagnant or pathogenic Qi that has been released during the analgesic stage. Apply striking techniques such as Ji fa and Pai fa and brisk, light techniques like Ma fa, whisking–sweeping and Ca fa. This stage helps to invigorate the patient and bring them back up into ordinary waking consciousness.

Sex		Age	

Main complaint/reason for initially seeking out treatment

Presenting signs and symptoms of main complaint

Secondary complaints

Presenting signs and symptoms of secondary complaints

Relevant background information

• History of disease

• Surgery/physical trauma

• Significant emotional events/trauma

Interesting visual observations

• Colors

• Posture

• Shen

Information revealed through initial palpation of:

• Local areas

• Related areas, channel sinews, primary channels and points

• Abdomen

Any other useful information picked up, for example:

• The sound of the patient's voice

• From their odor

• From what you sensed of their dominant emotional tones

Tongue

Pulse

Initial diagnosis

Treatment principle

First treatment
What is your general approach and intention?

Describe the initial treatment including:

• The points prescription and the techniques you will use to stimulate them

• The channels you will work on and how

• The progression of the treatment from one area of the body to another. Where will you start the treatment: on the back or front, on the affected side or the opposite side, locally or distally? Where will you progress to and where will you finish? How long will you spend on each area?

• The techniques you will use and how you will apply them. Will you use any of the foundation routines?

• Where will you direct your intention and Qi? At what level? Wei Qi, Ying Qi, Yuan Qi, Blood, Zangfu?

• Will you use any gua sha, cupping or moxa? If so, what, where, when and how will you apply these?

• Will you use any external massage media?

If this is a patient in clinic that you are working with continue with these questions:

During treatment did you feel and find anything significant as you worked that gave you further information or changed your mind about your diagnosis or approach?

How long was the treatment?

How did the patient respond to the initial treatment?

Subsequent treatments

Did you make any changes to your approach or diagnosis?

Fig. 10.1 Case format.

Work distally before locally

Open the channels in the limbs, feet and hands to create a clear passageway for dredging stagnant and pathogenic Qi out of the body. For problems in the upper body, use the arm channels for dredging. For problems in the lower half of the body, dredge through the leg channels. For example, if a patient has lower backache, open up the Bladder channel in the legs and stimulate relevant distal points first, then work on the upper back and gradually move towards the lower back to apply the local work.

If you are treating a Deficient condition, stimulate distal points and work along the relevant arm and leg channels with gentle techniques. For example, if a patient has Lung-Qi Deficiency, work along the Lung channel in the arm and stimulate distal points before doing any work on the chest.

Treat the healthy side first

This is particularly important in the treatment of one-sided pain, atrophy and muscular skeletal problems. By working on the healthy side of the body first, you are initially drawing the patient's attention to what is healthy. You are affirming and reminding the body of how it is in health and what it can return to. You are also working preventatively; as the channels are bilateral, it is quite common to see a channel sinew problem, for example, moving across the body to affect both sides. If, for example, a patient has tennis elbow on the right, work their left arm first for about half the amount of time you would spend working the affected side on the right.

Putting these general principles together, if a patient has lower backache on the left side, treat distally along the Bladder channel in the calf on the healthy right side first.

Treat the back (Yang) before the front (Yin)

Treating the back affects the whole body through the powerful actions of the channels and points that run through it. Whether you want to tonify Qi, nourish Blood, strengthen the functions of the Zangfu, or release the channel sinews, clear pathogens and move stagnation, Tui na treatment will generally involve some work on the patient's back.

Working the protected Yang side of the body first allows the patient to relax and yield. If you are treating respiratory, digestive and gynecological conditions, always work the relevant areas and points on the patient's back before working on the front in the Yin and more vulnerable areas of the chest and abdomen. For example, if a patient has menstrual problems, you would start treatment by working on the Governing Vessel and Bladder channel, stimulating relevant Governing Vessel, Back Shu and Huatuojiaji points and generally working on the lower back, sacrum and hips. You would then work distally in the leg channels before applying any abdominal treatment.

If you are working on a Yang channel sinew muscular skeletal problem, work on the Governing Vessel first which governs all Yang.

Feel, find and follow

If a patient has pain, discomfort or restricted joint movement, the first thing to do is to go to that painful place and touch it, feel it and explore it. Like a Tui na detective, find the Ah Shi points, the areas of tension, holding and restricted movement. Follow these areas of tension, adhesion, holding and so on by continuing to palpate the channel sinews along the course of the muscles, tendons and ligaments. Follow what you feel under your fingers and thumbs until the quality of the connective tissue changes.

Feeling, finding and following is a diagnostic tool as well as a form of treatment. Before any treatment begins it provides precise diagnostic information about the location, extent and nature of the problem and the channel sinews involved. When you arrive at the stage of treatment where you want to work locally, go back to what you felt and found and begin to treat the Ah Shi points, release and stretch the channel sinews, break up the adhesion, free the joints and dredge all of this released stagnation and accumulation out of the body through the Jing Well points. Working in this way you will get very reliable feedback from your hands about changes and releases occurring in the connective tissue and develop highly sensitive palpation skills.

Clear Excess before nourishing Deficiency

When treating mixed patterns of disharmony, concentrate on reducing and clearing any Excess during the first part of the treatment and then focus on nourishing and tonifying in the second half of the treatment. For example, if a patient has Qi stagnation and Blood Deficiency, move and invigorate the Qi first and nourish Blood second. In women with mixed patterns, work on moving Qi and Blood, clearing, dredging and releasing any Excess in the Yang second half of their menstrual cycle up to their period. Focus on nourishing Blood, tonifying Qi and supporting the Zangfu in the Yin post-menstrual phase and up to ovulation.

Dredging the channels

During the analgesic stage of treatment as you release accumulated stagnation of Qi, Blood and pathogenic factors, it is important to remember to clear what has been released by either bringing it to the surface where it can be dissipated or by dredging it through the channels of the limbs. Techniques that are particularly useful for dredging are Tui fa, Gun fa and compound versions of Rou fa and Na fa, especially kneading–grasping, kneading–pinching and pinching–grasping. Work along the course of the channel sinews to the Jing Well points. When you arrive at the fingers or toes, use Nian fa. As you work, imagine dredging and pulling the pathogenic Qi through the channels and out of the Jing Well points which act as doorways to the Exterior.

Apply gua sha and cupping before Tui na treatment

If you want to apply gua sha or cupping, always do this first; massage over the treated areas to help to disperse Qi and Blood and then continue with the rest of the treatment.

Treatment tips

- **Choose the main points prescription.** Keep in mind that points need to be stimulated for between 1 and 3 minutes on average with Tui na, so keep your main points prescription simple, perhaps four distal points and one or two local points.
- **Choose how to stimulate the main points.** Which techniques might have the most therapeutic benefit and how will you apply them in relation to your intention to tonify/strengthen/disperse/clear/release and so on?
- **Choose a few secondary points.** As you are working along affected channels or areas of the body, you might choose to go into these points to palpate or treat if it seems appropriate.
- **Decide on the channels that you want to treat and at what level.** For example, you might choose the leg Tai Yang channel sinew or the Spleen primary channel. This is important in terms of your choice of points, techniques and methods of application and also where you have your attention and focus.
- **Decide how to stimulate those channels.** Choose three or four appropriate techniques and decide how you will apply them according to the effect you want to have on your patient's Qi, Blood, Zangfu and so on and bear in mind the general principles of treatment.
- **Decide on which areas/zones of the body require treatment.** Can you use any of the area foundation routines as a basis for treatment? If so, are there aspects of the routine that you will need to focus on for longer? Will you need to add something to the routine to make it more effective? Will you need to take some parts out altogether?
- **Will you apply any ancillary therapies, gua sha, cupping or moxibustion?** If so, where will you apply them and at what stage of the treatment will you apply them?
- **Treatment time.** Roughly how long will you spend on each part of your treatment?

Nourishing Xu Deficiency and clearing Shi Excess

Choice of techniques

Most Tui na techniques are versatile and can be used to treat both Xu and Shi depending on your intention and how you choose to apply them. For instance, An fa and Rou fa can be applied to strengthen Deficient Qi or to disperse and move stagnant Qi.

Some techniques lend themselves more naturally to dispersing, invigorating, dredging, restraining or nourishing and so on. For example, Mo fa is gentle and warming so it is a good choice in cases of Deficient Cold and Yang Xu. It soothes the Qi, relaxes and calms the mind, and in so doing, helps to nourish Yin. Patients with Blood and Yin Deficiency benefit greatly from the application of Mo fa.

In contrast, striking techniques such as Ji fa and Pai fa are particularly suited to dissipation and invigoration.

As you explore working with the techniques, their therapeutic natures reveal themselves. Tui na is a tangible treatment; as a practitioner you can feel what the techniques are doing. When you dredge the channels, it should feel like you are dredging, and when you are nourishing, it should feel nourishing.

Application of the techniques

Having chosen what you feel will be the most appropriate techniques, the most important factor is how you apply the techniques and your intention. The general principles to keep in mind are:

The speed of application

- **Fast** application is Yang; it speeds up the flow of Qi and is used to invigorate and move Qi and Blood and to clear and dredge Excess.
- **Slow** application is Yin; it slows Qi down and is used to nourish Deficiency, and cool, calm and restrain Qi.

The force of application

- **Strong and vigorous** application is Yang; it will warm, move and invigorate Qi, and break up and disperse adhesions and accumulations, e.g. Yin accumulations such as Phlegm and Blood stasis.
- **Gentle** application is Yin and will soothe, calm and slow down the movement of Qi, relax the patient and nourish Qi and Blood.

The direction of application

- **Working against the flow of the channel** is used for purging, clearing and dredging Excess from the channels. Bear in mind which level of channels you are working with, i.e. primary channels, channel sinews, divergent channels, as the channel sinews and divergents all move up towards the head with the exception of the San Jiao divergent channel. This is one reason why, with Tui na, we often move towards the hands and feet to clear and dredge Excess; we are moving against the flow of the sinew and divergent channels towards the Well points which act as doorways for the release of obstructing pathogenic factors.
- **Working with the flow of the channel** is used for Deficient conditions, tonifying, nourishing and supplementing Qi, Blood, Yin and Yang. In this case we are generally following the flow of the primary channels.
- **Working in a clockwise direction** encourages Qi to gather inwards; this has the effect of drawing it into a point or area to nourish, tonify and supplement.
- **Working in an anti-clockwise direction** moves Qi out; this has the effect of dispersing, clearing, releasing stagnation, obstruction, etc.

The length of time of application

- **Working for a short period of time** with a technique on a point, or along a channel, is used for moving and clearing Excess.
- **Working for a long period of time** will have a tonifying, nourishing effect.

In treatment these principles are usually combined in some way. For example, if you have chosen Yi zhi chan tui fa as a point-stimulating technique and your intention is to move stagnant Qi then you would work quickly and vigorously for a short period of time (about 1 minute) directing the movement and the Qi against the flow of the channel. If you want to tonify then you would work gently and slowly, with the flow of the channel, and for a longer period of time (about 3 minutes).

An example

With the above principles in mind, let us say I have a patient who has poor digestion, dull epigastric pain and bloating from Stomach-Yin Xu. They are also producing some phlegm, which they are often clearing from their throat. I come to the conclusion that they are manifesting the phlegm in an attempt to hold onto some Yin to redress the balance. My main objective therefore is to nourish the Stomach-Yin and to support the Spleen-Qi. My secondary objective is to dissipate the phlegm from the chest.

To nourish Stomach-Yin and Spleen-Qi I work slowly and gently, moving with the flow of the Stomach and Spleen primary meridians and working for a relatively long period of time along the channels and on points using Mo fa, Tui fa, Rou fa and An fa. I work on the abdomen with Mo fa and Rou fa focusing on Zhongwan Ren12 and working gently and slowly in a clockwise direction for 10 minutes. At the same time, I apply Rou fa with my thumb in a clockwise direction to points on the Stomach and Spleen channels using my other hand. I then apply Tui fa to the Stomach and Spleen Back Shu points with my thumbs and then hold the points for about 3 minutes each. Finally I apply the coordinated technique whisking–sweeping and Ji fa/Pai fa to their shoulders and upper back, working briskly to disperse phlegm.

Yin and Yang styles of practice

As you can see from the above principles, Yang is fast, strong, vigorous and short and pushes against the flow, so generally speaking, using a Yang style will move, warm, invigorate, break up, disperse, clear and dredge. Yin is slow, gentle and still and goes with the flow, so a Yin style of practice is generally more suited to nourishing, cooling, calming, containing, relaxing, supplementing and tonifying.

Warming palm

Warming palm is a very effective way of nourishing an area that is Weak or Deficient. Its application is versatile, for example it can be applied at the level of the Zangfu to strengthen the Qi of the internal organs, to the eyes and ears to improve sight and hearing, and to joints, muscles and tendons that have been injured and are Deficient in Qi and Blood.

Method of application

Rub your palms together until they are scorching hot and place them on the area to be treated. Keeping the tip of your tongue on the roof of your mouth just behind your teeth, draw Qi down from the universe through Baihui Du20 and into your Dantian as you inhale. As you exhale allow the Qi to move from your Dantian up into your chest, down through your Pericardium channel and out through Laogong PC8 into the organ or area to be treated. Apply for between 3 and 10 minutes.

How do we affect Qi at different levels using Tui na?

There are some techniques that are particularly good at affecting Qi at different levels. These levels are: Wei Qi, Ying Qi and Yuan Qi.

Wei Qi

Wei Qi is superficial and unpredictable by nature. Techniques that have a circular motion, particularly Rou fa, are very effective for treating at the level of Wei Qi. The circling motion acts a bit like a tornado. If you want to expel pathogens and help Wei Qi to disperse, then apply Rou fa to points and along channels in an anti-clockwise direction quickly and vigorously, working towards the Jing Well points. If you want to support and strengthen Wei Qi then apply Rou fa in a clockwise direction, working more slowly and gently and towards the head.

Any of the compound techniques that involve kneading will be effective at the Wei Qi level. Kneading–nipping, for example, is well-known for its ability to strengthen Wei Qi. One way of achieving this is to apply kneading–nipping to the Governing Vessel, working in a clockwise direction with the flow of the channel from the coccyx towards the head. Gua fa also stimulates Wei Qi; vigorous, fast application will move and disperse it and moderate application will strengthen it.

Ying Qi

Ying Qi has direction and moves with the Blood; it is affected by stimulating the primary channels and luo vessels. In acupuncture, the needling technique lifting and thrusting is used to reach the Ying Qi level. In Tui na, Na fa, compound versions of Na fa, An fa, Yi zhi chan tui fa and Ji dian fa will produce the same effect. If you want to apply Na fa to treat Excess at a Ying Qi level, then concentrate on the lifting up aspect of the technique, imagining that you are pulling the Excess up from the Ying to the Wei level to be released. If you want to nourish, concentrate on the releasing aspect of Na fa; imagine throwing Qi into the Ying level. If you are applying An fa or elbow Ya fa, angle your thumb or elbow with the flow for nourishing and against the flow for clearing. Also, for nourishing, concentrate on stimulating the point with press and release An fa, pushing in deeply, softly and slowly from the Wei to the Ying level and then releasing gently back to the Wei level then pushing in again. For clearing Excess, think of drawing out from the Ying to the Wei level by applying the techniques quickly and strongly.

Yuan Qi

Yuan Qi derives from Essence; rooted in the Kidneys it moves through the eight Extraordinary Vessels. To affect Yuan Qi we need to apply techniques that will ripple through to the deepest levels. These techniques are essentially Zhen fa applied to points such as Yuan source points and points of the eight Extraordinary Vessels and to the areas of the lower back and abdomen to affect the Kidneys. Fast application of Yi zhi chan tui fa with strong intention to reach the Yuan level can be applied, and if you have developed your ability to direct your Qi and intention, then it is possible to reach the Yuan level by using An fa. This is achieved by depth of focus and intention rather than depth of pressure.

Working in this way is effective for treatment at the level of the *eight Extraordinary channels*. To affect the *divergent channels* work on moving the joints. Yao fa is one of the most effective techniques for the divergents along with Dou fa, Cuo fa, Ba shen fa and other passive movements. To affect the *luo channels* we need to bring Blood up to the surface. Use gua sha or techniques like nipping–grasping and Che fa at the luo points. To affect the *primary channels* we treat points with any of the point-stimulating techniques and guide Qi along the channels with techniques such as Tui fa and Rou fa. To affect the *channel sinews* we can work with a variety of techniques, and passive movements to release and dredge the channels.

Working with breath and visualization

There are many ways of using visualization and breath to help the effectiveness of treatment. Some possibilities for you to try follow.

Basic principles

Working with the patient's breath

- Asking your patient to breathe into the area you are working on brings their consciousness to that place which will help Qi to flow there. *Where the breath goes, the attention follows and the Qi flows!*
- When applying deeper techniques for the purpose of releasing, dredging and dispersing, such as strong An fa, Ya fa and some of the passive movements, especially Yao fa and Ban fa, press deeper and stretch further on the patient's exhalation and release on their inhalation.
- For cases when there is a lot of very stubborn stagnation, accumulation and holding, instead of releasing your pressure with the inhalation, you can maintain your pressure at the same level and ask your patient to breathe into your pressure. This can be very effective for abdominal work such as releasing the diaphragm and the eight doorways around the navel.
- Give space for the patient's breath. As you work, the patient's breath patterns can change. Be aware of this. For example, when Qi that is obstructed begins

to move the patient may naturally take a deeper breath. It is important to just allow the space for this and to recognize that when the breath changes the Qi has also changed.

Visualization and using your own breath

Keep reminding yourself to draw upon the infinite Qi of the universe rather than your own personal Qi store.

Drawing down universal Qi

You can apply this method whenever you want to bring Qi to an area that is depleted, or after you have dispersed stagnant or pathogenic Qi and you want to draw some vitality back to a previously obstructed area.

With the tip of your tongue at the roof of your mouth just behind your teeth, draw Qi down from the universe through Baihui Du20 and into your Dantian as you inhale. Imagine the Qi as a bright white light coming down from the stars. You could imagine the Qi of the pole star and the plough constellation coming together and then descending as a great pillar of light, just as you would in the five-element protection exercise on pages 7–9. As you exhale, visualize the Qi moving from your Dantian up into your chest, connecting with your heart and then flowing down through your Pericardium channel and out through PC8, or through the Well points at your fingers and thumbs and into the area or point to be treated.

Drawing Qi up from the Earth

In addition to drawing Qi down from the universe, you can also pull Qi up through your grounding roots into Yong quan KD1, up the Yin channels of your legs and into your Dantian. Allow the Qi from the universe and the Earth to mingle in your Dantian and then flow together up to your chest, down the Pericardium channel and out of your palms or fingers.

You can also just use Qi from the Earth; this can be useful if your patient feels a lack of stability, support and grounding.

Sun and Moon Qi

If you want to warm and tonify Yang Qi, inhale and visualize drawing down the Qi of the Sun into your Dantian. Imagine a Sun shining brightly in your Dantian, another in your heart and one in each palm. Exhale Sun Qi into the area to treated.

To cool and to nourish Yin, inhale and visualize drawing down the Qi of the Moon into your Dantian. Imagine a full Moon shining in your Dantian, your chest and in both palms. Exhale Moon Qi into the area to be treated.

Five elements

There are several possibilities. Working with your hands over the organs, the Back-Transporting points, Front-Collecting points and other points associated with the chosen elements, you can simply visualize drawing down Qi from the universe that holds the color vibration associated with the element you want to work with. For example, if you want to tonify the Metal element you could hold

推拿

Zhong fu LU1, the collecting point, with the palm of one hand and hold Taiyuan LU9, the source point, with the tip of your middle finger and visualize Qi as white light or mist coming into your Dantian and out through your palm and finger, filling the patient's Lung channel and moving into the lungs.

You can be even more creative and visualize something that represents the element as well as the color associated with it. For example, if you wanted to work with the Wood element you could bring one palm to hold Liv14, the front collecting point, and the other hand behind to hold BL18, the Back Shu point. So you are holding the right rib-cage and the patient's liver is between your hands. Visualize a forest of strong healthy trees between your hands. If Wood is in Excess you might imagine pruning some trees or even a bit of tree surgery! You get the idea.

If you are familiar with six sounds Qigong, you can work with the sounds. If you are brave, make the sounds vocally, if not then make the sounds internally as you visualize the associated color or other image representing the element.

This work is very creative and you can have a lot of fun with it. Ideally get your patients involved in the process as well; they can work with you during treatments and also on their own in between treatments.

Asking the patient to visualize and engage

For some patients, profound transformations can occur during the course of treatment. This is especially the case when the patient is in some way consciously engaged with the process. One way of encouraging this is to ask your patients to imagine or visualize colors and images associated with the five elements, while you do the same. Another way is, as you work on an area of muscular holding for example, ask your patient to bring their breath there and ask them if any images, thoughts, memories or feelings come to mind. As you work the muscles and channels with Tui na you can stimulate body memory and release emotional and energetic holding patterns. It is quite common during treatment for patients to remember old injuries and traumas that they had forgotten about. This can be a very powerful and transformative way of working.

Treatment length and frequency

In the traditional Chinese medicine hospitals in China, patients often come for treatment every day until they are better. Treatment is given in blocks or courses of treatment. Acute conditions are treated in blocks of 3–5 daily treatments with a break of 1–2 days between each treatment block. Chronic conditions are treated every other day in blocks of 10–15 treatments with a 2–3 day break between each treatment block. Each treatment lasts for approximately 30–40 minutes.

For Western practitioners and their patients, this way of working is usually impractical in terms of time and cost. Most complementary and alternative medicine practitioners are working within the one patient, one practitioner, one hour, once a week psychotherapy model. I suggest that you treat patients with acute conditions every other day if possible. In my experience, if patients are in a lot of pain, they are usually willing to come more frequently in order to treat the problem as quickly as possible. This way, acute problems can often be treated within a week or two. In chronic conditions, depending on your approach and style of practice, treat patients either once a week for an hour or twice a week for half an hour. Think of treatment in 6–10 week blocks. Assess the progress after every five treatments, and make any changes that seem necessary. Generally, chronic conditions will improve in the first block of treatments, however, a second and sometimes third block of treatments is often needed to create the necessary fundamental changes. As patients improve, space the treatments out so that eventually you are giving them maintenance treatments once or twice a month.

Some Chinese medicine practitioners are now beginning to explore other ways of working that are more similar to the Chinese hospital approach and may be more suitable for the type of treatment we are offering. In terms of Tui na, from what I have experienced and observed, working in teams in one large room is in many ways ideal for the practitioner and the patient. Potentially the work can be shared, the treatment times and costs can be cut down and patients can come more frequently for treatment.

Contraindications and cautions

Tui na is a very safe form of treatment when practiced proficiently within the context of the rationale of Chinese medicine and the general principles of practice. However, there are a few cautions and contraindications to be aware of. These are as follows:

- **During pregnancy.** Do not work on a woman's abdominal area during pregnancy or on her lower back until after the fifth month of pregnancy. After this time you can work gently and moderately on the lower back with the patient lying on her side. Sciatica is common in the third trimester of pregnancy and Tui na is very helpful for this.
- **Cancer.** Be very cautious when working with cancer patients. Do not massage the site of a malignant tumor. Strong vigorous Yang style techniques or passive movements are contraindicated. However, gentle subtle Yin style Tui na can be very helpful to cancer patients. It will help to relax the patient, calm the Shen and support their Qi. It can also help with the side effects of conventional treatment such as chemotherapy.
- **Fractures and open wounds.** It is contraindicated to treat patients with fractures in the early stages, open wounds and areas that are bleeding.
- **Acute infectious diseases.** It is contraindicated to treat patients who have, or you suspect might have, a serious acute infectious disease such as viral hepatitis, viral meningitis or tuberculosis.
- **Bleeding disorders.** It is contraindicated to treat patients with hemorrhagic disorders such as hemophilia or if you suspect any acute internal bleeding.
- **Serious mental/emotional disorders.** Be cautious when treating patients who are medicated for

serious mental and emotional disorders such as manic depression and schizophrenia. A big conflict can be created within a patient who is taking powerful antipsychotic medication and having treatment with Chinese medicine. The two approaches are so different that the patient's Qi can become confused and chaotic.

- **Skin diseases.** Do not work on the skin or apply any external massage media to patients with skin diseases such as psoriasis and eczema. Working over the patient's clothes and a Tui na cloth is safe and suitable for patients with this type of skin disease.

- **Osteoporosis.** Be cautious and work gently and moderately with patients who have osteoporosis. Do not apply strong vigorous Yang style techniques or passive movements.

Generally, if you are at all in doubt about treating a patient, then I advise you not to. Seek advice from colleagues and more experienced practitioners and refer patients to their GPs.

CHAPTER 11

Muscular skeletal ailments

In the UK, it is estimated that about a third of the population suffers with some type of muscular skeletal problem. In practice, these are some of the most common complaints that you will see. In my experience, about 80% of patients come with main or secondary complaints of muscular skeletal discomfort, tension, stiffness, pain, numbness or limitation of movement. Tui na is famous for its ability to treat muscular skeletal problems and for good reason; clinically it is highly effective and produces excellent results.

In this chapter I will give you suggestions, ideas and tips on how to approach the treatment of muscular skeletal problems. I will not give prescriptions for the many and varied ailments of this nature that you may come across; for this I suggest you refer to the Tui na books that have been compiled in China and translated into English (please see the recommend reading list at the end of this book).

My aim is to provide you with some structure and guidelines for an approach that can be applied in the treatment of a wide range of muscular skeletal ailments. I have included several cases to help to illustrate the treatment of common muscular skeletal ailments.

Some of the most common muscular skeletal problems that you are likely to see are:

- Lower backache
- Sciatica
- Arthritis and rheumatism
- Frozen shoulder
- Tennis/golfer's elbow
- Wry neck
- Repetitive strain injury (RSI)
- Carpal tunnel syndrome
- Chronic muscular tension and joint restriction
- Pain related to old traumas and injuries
- Sprains and strains from trauma/sports injuries

Bi syndrome (*painful obstruction syndrome*)

In Chinese medicine, most muscular skeletal ailments are due to Bi syndrome (*painful obstruction syndrome*). The normal healthy flow of Qi and Blood through the channels becomes blocked and causes pain, numbness, stiffness, aching and restricted movement of the muscles, tendons, ligaments and joints. The obstruction is caused by invading pathogenic factors, essentially Wind, Damp and Cold. In most cases all three factors are present, but one predominates.

In the case of Wind-Damp Heat or Hot Bi syndrome, the Heat is either a by-product of trapped stagnant Wei Qi, which when obstructed tends to produce symptoms associated with inflammation such as heat, swelling, nerve pain and severe pain, or from an internal disharmony such as Empty Heat from Yin Xu. When there are no obvious signs of pathogenic factors, then the obstruction is due to stagnation of Qi and Blood. This can be caused by many factors such as lack of exercise, overstrain and internal disharmony.

Bi syndrome can be acute or chronic and can affect the muscles, tendons, ligaments, joints and bones. When Bi syndrome affects the channel sinews, Tui na can usually treat the problem quite quickly. Chronic bony Bi syndrome that involves structural, bony changes, such as you might see in rheumatoid arthritis, will take a longer time to treat; other factors such as Phlegm and Blood stasis can be involved and need to be addressed.

All muscular skeletal problems have one thing in common – *stagnation*! It is just a question of figuring out what is causing the stagnation. The main causes are:

- Invading pathogenic factors
- Overstrain/overuse
- Lack of exercise
- Poor postural habits
- Emotional holding patterns
- Injuries/traumas
- Underlying Deficiency

Once you know the cause, you can treat at the appropriate level and advise your patients about any lifestyle changes, exercises, etc. that may help.

Treatment

Depending on your diagnosis, the treatment of muscular skeletal problems usually involves a combination of the following:

- Warming, relaxing and releasing the channel sinews (muscles, tendons and ligaments)
- Breaking up, dispersing and dredging stagnation, congestion and accumulation of Qi and Blood
- Breaking up and dispersing fibrous adhesions, caused by injuries, traumas, surgeries, etc.
- Moving and invigorating the flow of Qi and Blood
- Expelling, clearing, dispersing and dredging obstructing pathogenic factors from the channels
- Lubricating and facilitating the movement of joints
- Nourishing, tonifying and supporting Qi, Blood, Yin and Yang
- Bringing the patient's awareness and breath to areas of habitual holding and/or collapsing
- Encouraging and supporting relevant lifestyle changes

General tips and suggestions

- Take time to observe your patient's posture; what are your eyes drawn to? Put yourself in the same position, exaggerate it and feel what is happening in your body.
- Ask your patient to perform a range of movements relevant to the affected muscles, tendons and joints and observe what is happening in their body and which movements are restricted. This will help you to find which channel sinews are primarily affected.
- The first time you see a patient, spend a lot of time palpating. Palpate the areas where the patient feels pain. Feel, find and follow along the channel sinews searching for Ah Shi points, tension, adhesion, areas of Emptiness and Fullness, Heat and Cold. Palpate the whole of the affected channel for Ah Shi points.
- Discover the dominant pathogenic factor involved, if there is one. This will help you to choose which Tui na techniques to apply, which ancillary thera-

pies may be useful and which external massage media to use.

- In the treatment of chronic conditions where there is both Excess and Deficiency, clear the Excess factors first, move Qi and Blood, expel pathogens and dredge the channels and then nourish the underlying Deficiency in the second half of the treatment.
- Remember to treat distally as well as locally, for example, in neck problems, treat the forearm channels, and for lower back problems, work in the calf along the Bladder channel.
- If your patient is frail or the problem is either very chronic or connected to an old traumatic injury, especially one involving a break or fracture to the bone, consider working in a Yin style with your attention at the level of the bone.
- Follow the general principles of treatment given on pages 130–133.

Channel sinews

The biggest, most substantial channels in our bodies are the channel sinews or tendino-muscular meridians. They are the protective connective tissue armor of the body consisting collectively of muscles, tendons and ligaments. Wei Qi flows through the channel sinews, and in health, when Wei Qi is strong and unobstructed, the sinews are flexible, supple, supportive and strong, enabling us to function well and express ourselves in the physical world. If Wei Qi becomes obstructed or Deficient, the sinews become compromised, restricted, rigid, stiff, painful or weak and unsupportive.

Tui na has a special relationship with the channel sinews, after all it is the sinews that we are grasping, kneading, rolling, and so on. Tui na can work with the channel sinews in a number of powerful ways, and is extremely effective in the treatment of acute and chronic sinew Bi syndrome. As well as treating functional muscular problems, treatment of the channel sinews can effect and bring changes to the structure of the body. For example, in the case of scoliosis, it is possible to facilitate changes in the shape of the spine by working deeply to release the Bladder channel sinew. The channel sinews also deal with emotional armoring and working with them can lead to powerful emotional release.

From a clinical point of view, the Yang channel sinews are the most important and all acute muscular skeletal conditions can be treated via the leg and arm Yang channel sinews. In chronic cases there are other issues involved such as Blood Deficiency and Zangfu disharmonies, especially Kidney-Yin and Yang Xu, Spleen-Qi Xu, Liver-Qi stagnation and Liver-Blood Xu. In chronic cases the underlying disharmony must be addressed and the partner Yin channel sinew treated as well.

I encourage you to familiarize yourself with the pathways of the channel sinews in some detail; look at the places where they bind, meet and converge. Memorize the pathways by working along them with your Tui na techniques and by going through the area foundation routines. Feel as many healthy channel sinews as possible

Table 11.1 Areas where channels meet

Tai Yang	Shao Yang	Yang Ming	Tai Yin	Shao Yin	Jue Yin
BL11, BL41 Nape area	GB12, SJ17 Mastoid area	ST12 Clavicle area	LU1, SP20 Pectoral area	Ren22 Throat area	Liv14, PC1 4th–6th intercostal spaces

so that you know when something does not feel right, and when something is Full, Tight, congested, Empty, Weak and so on.

Channel sinew pathways

All channel sinews begin at the Jing Well points:
- **Leg Yang channel sinews** move up to the face and converge around the area of Juliao ST3
- **Arm Yang channel sinews** move up to the head and converge around the area of Touwei ST8
- **Leg Yin channel sinews** move up and converge in the abdomen around Shenque Ren3
- **Arm Yin channel sinews** move up and converge at Yuanye GB22

Palpation of the channel sinews

When patients come for treatment they describe what they feel and show you where they are feeling their pain, stiffness and aching. This essential information should immediately get you thinking about which channel sinew is affected. Once the patient has described the location and nature of their pain, you then need to feel the area. Palpate the channel sinew that you think is affected. Follow the principle of feel, find and follow, palpating along the channel sinew looking for Ah Shi points, areas of Fullness, Tightness, adhesion and congestion, for Heat and swelling, for places where Wei Qi is obstructed. Feel for Weak, Cold, Empty, numb areas where Wei Qi is insufficient. Palpate the areas where the arm and leg channels meet for tenderness; these are important areas to release in treatment. Although listed in Table 11.1 as points, think of these meeting places more as the whole area around the points.

Suggestions and tips for treating painful obstruction of the channel sinews

- Identify the channel sinew at the root of the problem. This is done through palpation and by discovering which movements are restricted or elicit pain.
- Stimulate the Ah Shi points that you found on palpation as you work along the affected channel. Rou fa and Yi zhi chan tui fa are excellent point stimulating techniques for channel sinew problems.
- Stimulate the Jing Well points of the affected channel sinew with strong Rou fa or direct moxa. Use the Well points as doorways to expel pathogenic factors, and to activate the movement of Wei Qi.
- For all Yang channel sinew problems, release the Governing Vessel first with gua sha and techniques like Gua fa, pinching–grasping, nipping–grasping and kneading–nipping.

- Stimulate the Huatuojiaji points with techniques like Yi zhi chan tui fa, Tan bo fa, An fa, Rou fa and Ji dian fa. For neck and upper limb problems, check the Huatuojiaji points from T1 to T7 for tenderness, tightness and so on and work on the most tender or congested areas. For lower back and lower limb problems, do the same with the points from T11 to L5.
- Release major areas around joints where the channel sinews bind with techniques like Gun fa, compound versions of Na Fa and Rou fa and Tan bo fa.
- Stimulate and release the areas where the channel sinews meet and converge.
- If there is adhesion and a lot of joint restriction, use Zhen fa, Ji dian fa, Tan bo fa and passive movements such as Ba shen fa and Yao fa to break up the adhesions and facilitate the movement of the joints.
- For problems of the leg yang sinews, release Quepen ST12 which is a major binding area. Gua sha is very useful to disperse obstructed Qi in this area.
- Dredge the channels with Gun fa, Tui fa and compound versions of Na fa and Rou fa.

For all muscular skeletal problems, the area foundation routines will provide a good framework for you to build your treatment around. Stimulate points and channels that are appropriate to the underlying disharmony with relevant techniques and methods. Remember to work on the good side as well as the affected side. For some further suggestions in the treatment of Bi syndrome see Table 11.2.

Chronic conditions

In chronic conditions it is essential to address the underlying internal disharmony:

For muscular weakness, atrophy and chronic fixed Bi syndrome, tonify the Spleen. Work along the Stomach and Spleen channels with Tui fa, Mo fa, gentle Gun Fa and Ca fa. Stimulate relevant points as you work along the channels. Work on the abdomen with techniques like palm Rou fa and tai chi Mo fa and stimulate the back shu points for the Stomach and Spleen with Rou fa and figure-of-eight Tui fa.

For problems with tendons and ligaments, chronic wandering Bi syndrome and patients who generally have very wiry muscles, move stagnant Liver-Qi and nourish Liver-Blood. This is common in women. Stimulate the four flowers BL17 and BL19 with moxa and then apply gentle Rou fa to the points. Work along the Liver channel with Tui fa, and Rou fa stimulating relevant points as you go.

For bony changes and deformities, nourish the Kidneys. Apply gentle Gun Fa to the lower back and palm Rou fa, Mo Fa and figure-of-eight Tui fa around the Kidney Back Shu points.

Table 11.2 Suggestions for the treatment of Bi syndrome

Signs and symptoms	Useful techniques/ancillary therapies
'Wandering Bi' Wind predominates	
Rapid onset of symptoms Rapid change in symptoms Pain that moves location Pain that involves several joints Pain that radiates Aversion to Wind Stiffness and pain in muscles and joints Possibly also fever, chills and other symptoms of an Exterior invasion (e.g. Floating, Superficial pulse)	Use gua sha along the Governing Vessel from Du16 to Du4, concentrating on the area of Du14, along the Bladder channel from BL10 to BL23 concentrating on the area of BL12 and at SI12 and ST12 If there is radiating pain, treat the place where the pain radiates to first with techniques like brisk anti-clockwise Rou fa and compound versions of Rou fa and Na fa and then work back towards the local area Yi zhi chan tui fa, Rou fa and nipping techniques are good for point stimulation
'Painful Bi' Cold predominates	
Signs of contraction and stagnation Severe biting or stabbing pain, often in only one joint Worse for cold and better for warmth No redness or feelings of heat Thin sticky white tongue coating Tight, Stringy, Wiry pulse	Direct moxa cones on the affected area, blowing the smoke as it burns to help to disperse the Cold. Yi zhi chan tui fa, Ji dian fa and Zhen fa for point stimulation Warm the Governing Vessel with Tui fa, Rou fa and Ca fa and the Bladder channel with Gun fa and Ca fa Gun fa around the Kidney Back Shu points Ca fa across Du4 and BL23 To increase Yang, apply lifting–grasping along the spine from the sacrum to the nape several times
'Fixed Bi' Damp predominates	
Pain in muscles and joints with a fixed location Heaviness in the affected area; a feeling that the area is tightly bound Stiffness and numbness more than pain Swelling Worse on cloudy, rainy, damp days Often affects the lower parts of the body Thick, greasy tongue coating Slippery, Soggy pulse	Apply indirect moxa with a stick to the local area Moderate cupping is also useful locally Gun fa on the affected area and along the related channels Pai fa and Ji fa on the limbs, back and local area to dissipate the Damp Ca fa on the legs along the Stomach and Spleen channels Strengthen the Spleen by stimulating BL20 with gentle Yi zhi chan tui fa and forearm or palm Rou fa. Work on the abdomen with Tui fa, Mo fa and Rou fa to strengthen the Spleen
'Hot Bi' Heat predominates	
Redness Hot to touch Inflammation Pain that is so bad the person cannot bear to be touched Rapid pulse Red tongue with yellow coating Possibly also other Heat signs (e.g. thirst, fever, irritability)	Apply gua sha first along the Governing Vessel from Du16 to Du4 and the Bladder channel from BL10 to BL23 Cupping on the Governing Vessel and Bladder channel is also useful Nipping–grasping along the Governing Vessel focusing on Du14, also along other relevant channels and to stimulate points such as LI11 and LI4 Hold the local area and focus on projecting Moon Qi for cooling at the end of the treatment

When treating chronic conditions, working with a Yin approach is very effective. Hold and connect the relevant points and direct Qi into the depleted organs.

Case studies

The following cases will help to illustrate how the above can work in practice. Tui na can have some quite remarkable results, even in very chronic cases where other forms of treatment have failed.

Lower backache

Main complaint

Julie, aged 42, had been suffering with chronic backache on and off for 7 years since the birth of her two children.

She constantly felt a low-grade dull ache and stiffness in the area of her sacrum. Over the previous 4 months the ache had become stronger and she was now experiencing some sudden intense shooting pains in her sacrum that radiated out across the right posterior superior iliac spine and down below her right buttock. These shooting pains were aggravated when she stood up from sitting and when she bent forwards. The aching and stiffness were worse in the morning when she got up and all the symptoms were better with warmth.

Julie is a vital and lively character who leads a very full life. She works in a demanding full-time job, is studying for a master's degree and is a keen runner and cyclist. She was still continuing to run and cycle because she said that although she ached afterwards, it did not make it any worse and that while she was exercising she felt better.

Palpation and observation

On palpation the tender points were BL28, BL54, BL36 and BL40. The whole sacral area felt Weak and Empty on palpation and the paraspinal muscles were the opposite – very Full and Tight, particularly around T11.

Secondary complaints

She also had aching knees and often felt stiff in the top of her shoulders. Other than this she was generally in very good health.

Tongue

Her tongue was a little pale.

Pulse

Her pulse was slow with a noticeable Emptiness in both root positions.

Diagnosis

Stagnation of Qi and Blood in the Bladder channel sinew caused by obstructing Cold and an underlying Kidney Qi Deficiency.

Treatment principle

This was to warm and dredge the Bladder channel, release the channel sinews, encourage Qi and Blood to move and warm and strengthen the Kidney Qi.

Treatment

Adaptive level

- Tui fa along the Governing Vessel from the coccyx to Dazhui Du14 and along the Bladder channel from Dazhu BL11 to Zhiyin BL67 until warm
- Coordinated kneading–grasping to the trapezius area at the top of her right shoulder and Rou fa with the heel of the practitioner's hand down the Bladder channel on the left. Repeated three times on each side

Analgesic level

- Kneading–nipping between each vertebra from Du14 to Du2
- Rou fa to BL67 opening the Jing Well points
- Gun fa working down the leg from Chengfu BL36 towards the ankle, paying attention to Weizhong BL40 on the way. When the channel was warm, I continued applying Gun fa with one hand while I stimulated BL36 with Ya fa and BL40 with An fa using my other hand. I worked the least affected left leg first and then the right
- Ya fa at BL54 plus elbow Rou fa as the point warmed up, then Tui fa to dredge the channel towards the Well point
- As I worked I discovered that there was a lot of tenderness in the gastrocnemius along the channel sinew in her calf muscles, so I worked to release this area with Rou fa and Na fa, paying attention to any Ah Shi points as I worked and often coming back to dredge the channel with Tui fa

- Using a little woodlock oil, I applied Gun fa to her sacrum and hip area and Rou fa to her back, releasing the paraspinal muscles particularly from T9 to L2 and stopping at Ah Shi points to release them with An fa, Rou fa and Ji dian fa. As with the legs, I worked along the least affected side first
- Continuing with Gun fa in the local area, I introduced forearm Rou fa to the Kidney Back Shu points and Mingmen Du4 with my other arm
- Rou fa and Na fa to release the iliacus and gluteus areas
- Kneading–grasping and Tui fa to dredge the channel

Dissipative level

- Ji fa along the Bladder channel from the nape to the ankle. Pai fa over the lower back, sacrum and buttocks. Then whisking–sweeping to her back and down her legs

Strengthening and warming Kidney Qi

- In practice, I prefer to release, clear and dredge obstruction and stagnation in the first part of the treatment and to do any tonification at the end
- Three large moxa cones on ginger to Mingmen Du4 and Shenshu BL23
- Three rice grain moxa cones on Taixi KD3
- Holding KD3 with the middle finger of one hand and Tui fa pushing in a figure-of-eight with the palm of my other hand around the kidneys
- Ca fa with red flower oil to the kidney area and sacrum until she felt heat moving down her legs

Progress and subsequent treatments

I gave Julie treatment twice in the first week, after which she was beginning to feel quite a bit better, the shooting pains only coming every now and then and with far less intensity. She then came for treatment once a week for a further 4 weeks. Subsequent treatments were similar to that described above with some variations in points, and as time went on I also gave more attention to her upper back and neck, releasing the areas where the channel sinew strongly binds such as the lattisimus dorsi area under the scapula and the area of Tianzhu BL10. Treatments were 1 hour in length. The shooting pains went after four treatments and by the sixth visit she was only experiencing the low level dull ache and some stiffness first thing in the morning. She commented at this stage that it was the best her back had been in years. I now see her once a month for maintenance and preventative treatment.

Sciatica

Main complaint

Paul, aged 34, came with lower backache and sciatica with pain running all the way down the back of his right leg to his ankle.

He runs his own plumbing business, working long hours, often in very cramped and awkward spaces. He also has to drive a lot. Paul's back problems started when he injured his back while working on a heavy plumbing installation job. This resulted in two prolapsed lumbar discs at L4 and L5 at the age of 27. He said that his back had never been the same since the injury and that he suffered with frequent bouts of sciatica and always had some type of backache. This original injury plus the nature of his work had weakened his lower back leaving him vulnerable to further problems.

He described the current pain as a very strong ache in his sacrum and right hip accompanied by an intense shooting pain down the back of his right leg which was particularly painful in his calf. It was aggravated by sitting for long periods of time and especially by driving and felt better when he was moving around. He said the whole of his back felt stiff, tense and generally uncomfortable.

Palpation and observation

When I examined Paul's back there was a scoliosis from T11 to L5 from right to left. The Huatuojiaji points were Full on pressure on the right and Empty on the left; they were also tender on the right. His whole back was very tense and there was pain on palpation at BL25, Yaoyan BL53, BL54, BL56, GB30 and GB29. I also found Ah Shi points in the gluteus medius and tensor fasciae latae on the right which elicited intense pain down the back of his leg to GB40.

Secondary complaints

He had also suffered with piles for several years which had been bothering him more since this bout of sciatica.

Tongue

His tongue had a slightly purple hue.

Pulse

His pulse was Full and Wiry.

Diagnosis

Invasion of Wind-Cold leading to stagnation of Qi in the Bladder and Gallbladder channel sinews. Weakness of the Governing Vessel was an important factor which may have begun with the prolapsed discs at age 27. The Governing Vessel is intimately connected to Tai Yang and Wei Qi, so if over time it is not able to motivate Tai Yang, then problems can easily occur along the course of the channel sinew which becomes prone to repeated invasions of pathogenic factors. From here, the problem can easily move across to the Gallbladder channel sinew at the places where they bind such as around GB30 and the greater trochanter. The piles and scoliosis also alerted me to the involvement of the Governing Vessel.

Treatment principle

Open and strengthen the Governing Vessel, expel pathogenic factors, warm and dredge the Bladder and Gallbladder channel sinews, activate the circulation of Qi and Blood, and stop pain.

Treatment

Ancillary therapies

Cupping To relax the muscles and begin to move the Qi and Blood I applied 10 glass cups to his back along the Bladder channel starting at BL12 and also over GB30 and BL54, and an Ah Shi point in the gluteus medius. I used a fairly strong suction and left them in place for 15 minutes.

While the cups were in place I opened the Governing Vessel using Yi zhi chan tui fa on SI3 on the left and BL62 on the right. I then held the two points with my middle fingers and imagined them connecting, bringing my attention and Qi to the Governing Vessel.

I also worked on his legs, warming and dredging the channels using Tui fa, Rou fa, holding–grasping and Gun fa down the Bladder and Gallbladder channels. I then removed the cups and continued with the treatment.

Adaptive level

- Using a little woodlock oil I applied Tui fa and Rou fa to his back where the cups had been

Analgesic level

- An fa and compound versions of Na fa down his legs along the Bladder and Gallbladder channels
- Elbow Ya fa to BL36 and BL37 until the points became very warm and a strong sensation of Qi was felt. Ji dian fa was applied to BL40 at the same time
- Ya fa working deeply in the gastrocnemius, waiting for warmth and asking him to breathe into the sensation which was very strong. At the same time I applied kneading–grasping to BL60 and KD3 and pinching–grasping along the channel to BL67
- Tui fa, Na fa and Ji dian fa to dredge and disperse down the leg channels
- Kneading–nipping with my thumb tip at each intervertebral space to clear the Governing Vessel
- Ca fa down the Governing Vessel
- Double-handed Gun fa down the Bladder channel from the top of the shoulders to the waist
- Compound versions of Na fa and Rou fa to release areas of Fullness around the latissimus dorsi, nape and neck, concentrating on the areas where the channel sinew binds
- Elbow Tui fa several times down either side of the spine along the Huatuojiaji points
- Gun fa over the lumbar area, sacrum and buttocks in combination with elbow Ya fa or thumb An fa at local Ah Shi points and Huatuojiaji points at the same time
- Compound versions of Na fa and Rou fa to release the sacrum, gluteus and iliacus areas
- Strong Ya fa to the Ah Shi point in the gluteus near the posterior superior iliac spine which radiated pain to the ankle
- Tui fa to dredge the channels
- Thumb Rou fa to release the sinew around his ankle
- Rou fa to BL67 to open the Well point

Dissipative level

- Na Fa and Pai fa along the channels

Passive movements

- Yao fa to both hips, Ban fa as an end-of-range twist, while in the twist I applied Ya fa and Rou fa to GB29 and the piriformis area
- Ca fa with woodlock oil to his sacrum and hips

Progress and subsequent treatments

Paul came back for his second treatment 3 days later. The day after his first treatment the pain became very intense. The following day he began to feel a lot better. The intensity of the pain had decreased and the sciatic pain now only reached the back of his thigh. This initial aggravation of symptoms in my experience is a very positive sign, indicating that the obstructed Qi has begun to move. Patients who have this reaction often respond relatively quickly to treatment.

The second treatment followed along the same lines as the first. Cupping was applied only to his sacrum and right hip as the rest of his back was still marked from the cupping 2 days earlier. I spent longer focusing on the Huatuojiaji points from T11 to L5 using thumb An fa, elbow Ya fa and Ji dian fa on the right side which was Full and tense while simultaneously working along the leg channels. I also applied dispersing moxibustion by applying direct moxa cones to the two main Ah Shi points in the local area and blowing on the cones as they burnt. This method helps to disperse Cold.

When Paul came for his third treatment 4 days later he had no more sciatic pain. He was now only aware of an ache in his sacrum and right hip which he said was 50% less than it had been when we first started treatment. On examining his back, I noticed that his spine was much straighter and generally his whole back looked and felt more comfortable. I could still create a strong shooting pain down his leg when I applied pressure to an Ah Shi point in the gluteus medius so I continued to treat him twice a week for a further 2 weeks.

Treatment continued as above, working with the Huatuojiaji points and direct moxa. I worked strongly in the back of the thigh at the site where the pain radiated to before applying the local work. At the end of his third week of treatment, Paul's spine had realigned (the magic of the Huatuojiaji points) and I could no longer produce the shooting pain down his leg by pressing the Ah Shi point. He felt no more aching in his hip or sacrum. I showed him some simple back exercises to practice at home. Because of the nature of his work I suggested that I see him once a month for maintenance treatment, which I have done since then.

Frozen shoulder

Main complaint

Susan, aged 54, had been experiencing pain and restricted movement of her right shoulder for 6 months when she came for treatment. Her doctor had diagnosed frozen shoulder. The pain, which she described as severe, and the restriction of movement had become gradually worse and she was now finding it extremely difficult to brush her hair, fasten her bra and generally to dress. The pain was very severe at night and therefore disturbing her sleep. She was also experiencing some numbness and pins and needles in her hands. She said she always had cold hands but they were much worse since she developed the shoulder pain. She explained that the pain had started around the top of her scapula, nape and the back of her shoulder and had gradually crept around to both the front of her shoulder and upper arm and under her shoulder blade to her armpit and the sides of her ribs. The pain was not affected by the weather.

Palpation and observation

Observing Susan's posture, the first thing I noticed was that everything looked tight and held. She was holding her arms in to the sides of her body, her shoulders were raised, her upper back looked very tight, and she was collapsing her chest. On testing the range of movement of the joint, there was pain and considerable restriction of movement on external rotation and abduction. Palpation revealed Fullness and tenderness at the Huatuojiaji points from T1 to T7 on the right; especially tender were those at T3, T4 and T5. Other very tender points were BL15, SI15, SI12, SI11, SI9, SI5, HT1, GB22, LI11 and ST12.

Secondary complaints

Susan had always had good health and lots of energy up until 9 months previously when she started to experience gripping, dull chest pain, palpitations, pain down both arms and breathlessness on exertion. Her doctor thought she might have angina and sent her for an angiogram which came back normal. She told me that she thought stress was the cause of her problems. She said she knew that she probably pushed herself too hard.

Tongue

Her tongue was pale purple and had scallops.

Pulse

Her pulse was Weak and Deep.

Diagnosis

This was an interesting case of Xu Deficiency leading to Shi Excess. Susan's frozen shoulder was due to painful obstruction from Qi and Blood stasis. Wei Qi was obstructed primarily in the Tai Yang channel sinews, and also the Liver channel sinew, leading to pain, compromised movement of the joint, tension and Fullness of her upper back and scapula area and tenderness at the Huatuojiaji and Small Intestine points. The Small Intestine divergent channel was also involved. Obstructed Wei Qi was unable to move Blood. This divergent channel is associated with the ability to move Blood. SI10 where the divergent channel emerges was particularly tender; this point, which is strongly associated with Blood, can be used to move Blood into the sinews. The divergent channel also enters the axilla and comes out at GB22, the sinew channels' confluent point, also referred to as the great luo in some traditions. The Small Intestine divergent channel as we know enters the heart.

Chest pains, palpitations and breathlessness or chest painful obstruction preceded Susan's shoulder problems. These symptoms were caused by Heart- and Spleen-Yang Deficiency, which is reflected in the pulse and tongue. Insufficient Yang led to lack of movement of Qi and Blood and eventually Blood stasis. The Small Intestine divergent channel has attempted to deal with the Blood stasis and this in turn has affected the channel sinews.

This is a good example of how an internal Xu can lead to an Exterior Shi and how the divergent channels divert problems away from the important internal organs to the Exterior.

Treatment principle

This was to warm, relax and release the affected channel sinews, move and invigorate the flow of Qi and Blood through the channels, and tonify and warm the Heart- and Spleen-Yang.

Treatment

The initial three treatments focused on moving Qi and Blood and releasing and relaxing the sinews.

Ancillary therapies

I applied gua sha along the Governing Vessel and the Bladder channel, from Du14 across the top of the shoulder to ST12, across the Bladder channel at the level of BL15 and at SI10. I did this bilaterally. The sha that came to the surface was pronounced and dark purple, especially on the right.

Adaptive level

- Using red flower oil I applied Tui fa and Rou fa along the Governing Vessel, Bladder channel from nape to waist and Small Intestine channel from SI17 down to the Well point SI1.

Analgesic level

- An fa, Rou fa and Ji dian fa to the Huatuojiaji points
- Then I worked along the Small Intestine channel sinew towards the Well point, working with compound versions of Rou fa and Na fa and stimulating the following points as I worked: first SI1 with strong anti-clockwise Rou fa then SI15, SI12, SI11, SI10, ST12 and LI15 with anti-clockwise Rou fa and press and release style An Fa, concentrating on drawing Qi up to the Wei Qi level, stirring it up and getting it moving
- Zhen fa on SI10 and BL15 to move Blood
- Double-handed Gun fa to the nape and upper back for about 10 minutes
- Sliding Tui fa along the Huatuojiaji points from nape to waist using my elbow

Passive movements

I asked Susan to sit on a chair and applied:

- Yao fa and Ba shen fa several times to all the joints of the upper limb
- In between each round of Yao fa and Ba shen fa, I went back to releasing the channel sinews with Gun fa and compound Na fa and Rou fa techniques

Dissipative level

- Ji dian fa to the upper back, concentrating on the Bladder channel and the Huatuojiaji points
- Pai fa to the shoulder and scapula plus whisking and sweeping down the upper limb
- Dou fa and Cuo fa to the upper limb, and Ca fa along the Huatuojiaji points, the top of the

shoulders, the shoulder joints and down the Yang channel sinews

I worked on both arms and on the unaffected side for half the amount of time as the affected side.

Advice to the patient

I showed Susan some self-massage to apply to her forearm and to SI1 and SI5. I also recommended that she rotate all the joints of her upper limb six times in both directions and showed her some shoulder stretches and recommended that she did them twice a day.

Progress and subsequent treatments

Susan had a strong reaction to the first two treatments that involved headaches, nausea, palpitations and a pounding sensation in the sternocleidomastoid area of her neck. I had warned her that she might experience some symptoms during the initial stages of treatment as the obstruction began to disperse and the Blood to move. She was very good-humored about these unpleasant effects and also reported that the pain in the scapula area had been much better.

After the third treatment she had no further unpleasant effects and she was pleased to tell me that she had experienced no chest pain or breathlessness when running to catch the bus. At this stage she was able to abduct her arm quite well and generally the range of movement had increased.

On the fourth treatment I began to add the use of moxa. I applied three cones bilaterally to BL15 and BL20 and three to LI11 on the right. I also stimulated HT1 with the compound technique pushing–pressing GB22 and Ren17 with Zhen fa.

When I saw her for the fifth treatment she told me that she had had no pain for 3 days after treatment and had loads of energy so she had mowed the garden and run around doing things. That night the pain returned and was severe. I continued treatment as before, twice a week, including the moxa, and at the end of treatment worked gently in her chest with Tui fa, Mo fa and Rou fa. Finally I held HT5 and Ren14 with my middle fingers, with the intention of tonifying and warming.

After a total of 10 treatments Susan had full range of movement and was pain free. She was also running for the bus and generally running around in her life again without any breathlessness or chest pain. I continued to treat her once a fortnight until her pulses felt stronger.

Repetitive strain injury (RSI)

Main complaint

Gordon, aged 43, was suffering with pain in his left elbow and forearm. He told me that it was his work that was causing the problem. He worked as a theater electrician and every day his job involved him winding up and holding onto long electrical cables. He was right-handed so he wound the cable with his right hand over his left forearm which held the weight. He said that work had been very busy over the past few weeks with a new production coming in to the theater and it was due to carry on like this for another week. He said that when he tried to lift and hold weight, the pain was strong and intense in his elbow around the area of LI11 and radiated along the Large Intestine channel sinew to the middle of his forearm.

What was bothering him even more than the pain was the numbness, pins and needles and weakness he had started to experience over the previous 10 days in his left hand. The numbness was affecting mainly his thumb, index and middle fingers. He was very concerned that he would not be able to carry on working. He said that he had also noticed that he was starting to get some pain in his right elbow as well.

Palpation and observation

On palpation I found that Gordon's Large Intestine channel sinew was incredibly Full, Wiry and Tight from his elbow to his wrist in both arms and especially on the left. There was marked tenderness at LI11, LI10, LI6 and LI5. There was a significant area of stuck adhesion in the flexor carpi radialis around LI6 and wrist flexion and rotation were impeded. I also noticed that Gordon's left shoulder was raised.

Secondary complaints

He said that he also constantly had tight shoulders around the trapezius area. Otherwise he said he felt okay.

Tongue

His tongue was reddish purple with a redder tip.

Pulse

His pulse was Wiry and slightly Quick.

Diagnosis

The diagnosis was sinew Bi syndrome affecting the Large Intestine channel sinew. The repetitive overuse of the sinew had created stagnation and obstruction in the flow of Qi and Blood which were now unable to flow freely to the extremities. The Large Intestine channel sinew binds at SI12 and wraps around the scapula which is why he was experiencing the tightness in his shoulders. His tongue and pulse reflected Heat and stagnation which made me think that he was probably more stressed than he was either aware of or wanted to tell me about.

Treatment principle

This was to release, relax and dredge the Large Intestine channel sinew, disperse adhesions and obstructions, and encourage the smooth flow of Qi and Blood.

Treatment

I started treatment with Gordon sitting forwards on a chair. Initially I applied gua sha along the Governing Vessel, paying particular attention to Du14. In practice, I have found that in the case of any Yang channel sinew problem, it is very effective to activate and release the Governing Vessel first before working on the affected channel. I followed this with nipping-grasping and Ca fa.

Adaptive level

- Tui fa, Rou fa and Ca fa with woodlock oil to his back along the Bladder channel, across the tops of

his shoulders and scapula and along the Large Intestine channel sinew of both arms

Analgesic level

- Gun Fa to the tops of his shoulders and upper back focusing on the areas where the channel sinew binds and attaches; this area was very tender the first time I treated him
- While continuing to perform Gun fa with one hand on his right shoulder, I also began to work along the channel sinew in his arm with compound versions of Na fa; I repeated this on the affected left side
- Strong An fa to the Huatuojiaji points on both sides from T1 to T7 where the channel sinew attaches, adding Rou fa to the pressure for further stimulation; I did the same with SI12
- I then asked Gordon to lie down on his back and applied Gun fa along his Large Intestine channel sinew from LI15 to LI5 until his arm felt really warm
- I then released the major binding areas for the channel sinew at LI15, LI11 and LI5 and the area of adhesion that I had discovered during my initial palpation by using kneading and grasping and Tan bo fa
- I stimulated the Ah Shi points that I had found with Yi zhi chan tui fa and Ji dian fa then opened the Well point by kneading with my thumb nail
- I then dredged the channel with pinching–grasping and Tui fa
- Nian fa to all of his fingers several times

Passive movements

- Yao fa to his shoulders, wrists and fingers and Ba shen fa to his shoulders, elbows, wrists and fingers

Dissipative level

- I applied Cuo fa to his arms and the palms of his hands
- Ca fa with woodlock oil to finish

Advice to the patient

I gave Gordon a bottle of woodlock oil and suggested that he massage his forearms to warm up the muscles and get the Qi moving before he started work. I showed him how to stimulate the tender points in his forearms with Rou fa and suggested that he did that twice a day.

Progress and subsequent treatments

I saw Gordon again 3 days later and his symptoms were already 80% better. He looked incredibly relieved. On palpation there was a major change in the quality of his muscles which now felt softer and more pliable. The obstructed area around LI6 had dispersed and he told me that he had no more sensations of pins and needles and numbness. I gave him another treatment as above. He was due to work out of London so we did not arrange any further treatments at that point. I asked him to ring me and let me know how he was getting on, which he did about a month later; he told me that after the second treatment he had experienced no further problems. I did not see him again for 18 months when he returned with similar symptoms; this time he needed just the one treatment.

Fixed Bi syndrome of the knee

Main complaint

Joan, aged 75, had been suffering with knee problems for the previous 5 years and was finding it increasingly difficult to get up the stairs and to walk for any distance. Her doctor had told her it was arthritis and had prescribed painkillers, which did not help. Joan said her knees ached and felt very stiff, weak and heavy. They were worse in the morning and when the weather was damp.

Palpation and observation

Joan's knees were swollen and quite cold to touch, she felt sore along the Stomach and Spleen channel sinews in her legs and there was marked tenderness at SP9, ST35 and ST34.

Secondary complaints

Joan also complained of poor digestion; she said she felt bloated and uncomfortable in the epigastric area after eating and often had heartburn. This had been getting gradually worse over the last few years. The doctor had suggested she take Gaviscon. She also told me that she was often 'very mucusy' in her sinuses and chest. Joan had enjoyed very good health all her life and was a keen cyclist in her younger years. She had always had good energy but since the knee started to worsen she had been feeling very tired and a little depressed in spirits.

Tongue

Her tongue was slightly swollen and wet with some scallops at the sides. The tongue coating was peeled and shiny in the center and there were several horizontal cracks in the Stomach area.

Pulse

Her pulse was Weak and Slippery. Her Stomach pulse was especially weak.

Diagnosis

The diagnosis was Wind-Damp-Cold Bi syndrome with Damp predominant. There was underlying Spleen-Qi and Stomach-Yin Xu.

Treatment principle

This was to dredge and clear the obstructing Wind-Damp Cold from the leg channels, warm the channels, tonify Spleen-Qi and nourish Stomach-Yin.

Treatment

Adaptive level

* To open and warm the channels I applied Tui fa and Rou fa down the Stomach and up the Spleen channels of the legs

Analgesic level

I wanted to begin to do some supportive, tonifying work for Joan's Stomach and Spleen so I decided to apply coordinated techniques so that I could work the leg channels and the belly at the same time:

* Gun fa along the Stomach channel, working down from ST31, warming, dredging and motivating the Wei Qi; at the same time, I used clockwise Mo fa and then palm Rou fa at Zhongwan Ren12; I worked like this for about 10 minutes, with 5 minutes Gun fa on each leg
* Using Rou fa, I worked along the Stomach and Spleen channels, stopping to stimulate ST34 and ST35 with Yi zhi chan tui fa, ST36 with thumb Rou fa, SP3 with thumb Rou fa and SP9 with Yi zhi chan tui fa

Indirect moxa using a moxa stick over both knees for 5 minutes on each knee.

Dissipative leve

* Na fa, Pai fa with a hollow palm and a loose fist along the Stomach and Spleen channels
* Ca fa either side of her knees with a little dong qing gao

Tonifying

With the intention of supporting the Earth element, nourishing the Stomach and strengthening the Spleen I applied the following methods with my attention directed towards the level of the Zangfu:

* Joined palm Mo fa to the abdomen working in a clockwise direction
* Holding Ren12 and ST36 with middle fingers
* Holding the Stomach and Spleen with one hand over Ren12 and the other over Liv13 on the left side

I asked Joan to think of something that represented stability, strength and support, and to imagine that image between my hands. I worked with her like this for about 10 minutes.

Advice to the patient

Joan was very keen to help herself in any way possible so I showed her some simple self-massage to apply to her abdomen and taught her the Qigong healing sound for the Stomach and Spleen. We also discussed some dietary changes. She was a fan of cheese, drank quite a bit of milk and had a very sweet tooth. I encouraged her to try green tea, and to experiment with removing cheese and milk from her diet for the next month. I also encouraged her to eat her carbohydrates at breakfast and lunchtime and not to eat them as snacks later in the day or for dinner. Her digestive symptoms were always worse in the evening and I thought it might be beneficial if she gave the Stomach- and Spleen-Qi less work when it was at its lowest ebb.

Progress and subsequent treatments

Joan came for treatment once a week for 10 weeks and made steady progress over this time. I continued to work in a similar manner to that described above, sometimes adding the following work on her back to strengthen the Wei Qi and to further support the Stomach and Spleen:

- Using toasted sesame oil I applied Tui fa along the Governing Vessel from the coccyx to the nape and along the Bladder channel, working with both hands down the back to the sacrum
- Forearm Rou fa over BL20 and BL21 and Gun fa along the Bladder channel of the leg, focusing for longer at the popliteal fossa
- Thumb Rou fa to stimulate BL20 and BL21
- Pai fa along the back and down the backs of the legs
- Ca fa along the Governing Vessel and across the Stomach and Spleen Back Shu points
- Finally, holding the back of the knee with my Laogong focused at BL40 with one hand, while the other hand applied Tui fa in a figure-of-eight around the Stomach and Spleen Back Shu points; this was repeated on both sides

By the end of the 10-week course of treatments, Joan's knees were feeling stronger, she was able to walk without discomfort and the stiffness and heaviness were about 75% better. She also reported improvements in both energy levels and digestive symptoms. She was a very cooperative patient and willingly took on the dietary changes and self-massage which she felt were helping a great deal.

I continued to treat Joan on a fortnightly basis for a further six treatments and the improvements continued. Joan is now a sprightly 78-year-old woman with a new-found interest in nutrition. She comes to see me occasionally, usually in the winter, if she feels any return of her original symptoms.

Cervical spondylosis (a case from my colleague Weishe Song)

Main complaint

Fred, aged 76, had been suffering with chronic neck pain for 15 years after a car accident. He constantly felt a stabbing pain and stiffness in his neck and trapezius area, more on the left than on the right side. Over the previous 10 months the pain had become gradually worse. His doctor sent him for an X-ray after which he was diagnosed with nerve root type cervical spondylosis affecting C4–C5, C5–C6 and C6–C7. He was prescribed some very strong painkillers that did not make any difference. Fred's pain got worse when he kept the same position for too long or when it was cold and it improved a little when it was warm. His left hand felt numb all the time.

Palpation and observation

The back of his neck was very flat, the natural curve having almost entirely disappeared. His range of movement was very compromised at about 25% of what it should be in forward flexion, backward extension, side flexion and rotation. His ligamentum nuchae and trapezius muscles were stiff and hard. The tender points were GB20, GB21, SI13 and vertebral gaps between C5–C6 and C6–C7.

Secondary complaints

He also suffered from headaches, which manifested mainly in his left temple area. He felt tired all the time and had cold hands and cold feet. He had no history of hypertension or diabetes.

Tongue

His tongue was slightly pale with a thin coating and a few dark purple spots on the tip of the tongue. The veins under the tongue were swollen and dark purple.

Pulse

His pulse was Wiry and Deep in both rear positions.

Diagnosis

The diagnosis was Bi syndrome due to stagnation of Blood and an underlying Kidney-Yang Deficiency.

Treatment principle

This was to warm and dredge the neck channels, clear stagnation and strengthen Kidney-Yang.

Treatment

Adaptive level

After explaining to Fred the purpose of the treatment:

- Tui fa with my thumbs along the Gallbladder, Bladder and Governing Vessel channels from the bottom of the occiput all the way down to C7 level; each line was stimulated for 2 minutes
- Rou fa with my thenar eminence along the side of the neck for 5 minutes

Analgesic level

- Gun fa along either side of the neck and the top of the shoulders for 10 minutes
- An Fa and Rou fa with my right thumb in between each vertebra from C1 to T1 for 10 minutes
- Yi zhi chan tui fa on the following points, 2 minutes for each point: Tai Yang (extra), GB20, GB21, SI11, SI3, LI4
- Tan bo fa on HT1 (left side) for 1 minute until a tingling feeling moved down his arm
- Na fa to the nape and the top of his shoulders for 2 minutes
- Yao fa and Ba shen fa on his neck and shoulder, twice on each area
- Dou fa to both shoulders

Dissipative level

- Ji fa to the sides and back of his neck and across the tops of his shoulders for 3 minutes
- Pai fa with a hollow fist to his shoulders and upper back for 3 minutes

Tonifying Kidney-Yang

Having finished the neck treatment, I applied Zhen fa with both palms on his Dantian area until he felt warm in the whole abdominal region; then I applied Ca fa on his lower back and sacrum until it was very hot.

Advice to the patient

I suggested that Fred should look after his neck by keeping it warm, especially in cold weather, and I showed him some simple Qigong exercises for his neck. I taught him how to apply self-massage to GB20, GB21, LI4, LI10 and PC6 every day and I also encouraged him to go to the local tai chi class.

Progress and subsequent treatment

Fred came for treatment once a week for 5 weeks and made great progress over this period. The pain was much relieved and his range of movements gradually increased. He even drove to France for a 1-week holiday, which would have been impossible in the past.

His other symptoms like tiredness, headache and numbness in the left hand also improved a great deal. But his cold hands and cold feet remained the same. I taught him to apply moxibustion using a moxa stick, bird-pecking style. I asked him to apply this technique to Ren4 once a day for 10 minutes each time to reinforce Yuan Qi and strengthen Kidney-Yang.

I carried on treating Fred on a fortnightly basis for a further five sessions and the improvements continued. After applying self-moxibustion treatment for 5 weeks, his hands and feet started to warm up and his energy levels really began to increase.

He continues to see me once a month.

CHAPTER 12

Digestive disorders

Common digestive disorders

Many patients who come for Tui na treatment have digestive problems as part of their presentation. Common complaints include:

- Irritable bowel syndrome (IBS)
- Constipation
- Diarrhea
- Epigastric pain
- Abdominal pain
- Acid reflux
- Belching and flatulence
- Hypochondriac pain
- Poor appetite

Factors in common digestive disorders

The causes of these ailments are generally a combination of factors such as dietary inadequacies and excesses, irregular eating patterns, overwork and stress. Any combination of these lifestyle factors can lead to deficiency of Qi, Blood, Yin and Yang and to stagnation of Qi and accumulation of Heat, Cold and Damp.

Other factors in common digestive disorders

The small intestine

Sometimes known as the abdominal brain, the small intestine sits at the foot of the heart, sifting and sorting, absorbing what is useful, and passing on what is not to the large intestine and bladder to be excreted. This applies to thoughts and emotions as well as to nutrients. If you practice in a big city as I do, patients often report feeling overwhelmed, having too much to do, too much work, not enough time to reflect; they feel pushed by the general energy around them and find it very difficult to relax. Generally, there is a feeling of being hyperstimulated. In attempting to deal with all of this mental and emotional energy information, the small intestine, and consequently the large intestine, can become tense, tight and knotted, much in the same way as our shoulders develop tension and congestion when we are stressed and pushing our Qi too hard.

On palpation, the small intestine should feel soft and move easily and painlessly; often however, it feels tight, knotty and uncomfortable on palpation. As well as affecting the digestion, knotted and compromised intestines can lead to various problems such as menstrual disorders, emotional problems and back pain. Tui na is very effective for releasing these areas of stagnation and accumulation.

Suggested methods for releasing stagnation of Qi manifesting as accumulation, adhesion and knotting in the abdomen

The abdomen is a sensitive area and this work can get quite deep and be a bit uncomfortable both physically and emotionally. Always start by working initially on the patient's back and chest. Old traumas can be held in the small intestine, particularly around the navel, and powerful release work can be done by freeing up the accumulated and stagnant emotional Qi. The following method is suggested:

- Start with Mo fa using the pads of your index, middle and ring fingers. Work from the navel out in small anti-clockwise circles.
- Moving slightly deeper, work in the same manner as above using Rou fa, feeling for areas of knotting, tightness and congestion and asking your patient to let you know of any tender or painful areas. Apply this three times.
- Go back to the knotted areas that you found and begin to disperse them with fast anti-clockwise Rou fa, Zhen fa and Ji dian fa.
- With both palms over the area of the small intestine, apply Rou fa in a wave-like motion, as if rolling a ball that is inside the patient's belly, between your hands.
- Bring the ulnar edge of your palms to beneath the patient's ribcage, fingers just below the sternum, and use Rou fa to release the diaphragm, thinking of drawing it down towards the navel.

The navel

Ren8 – 'spirit door' – is a place that can provide an exit for stagnant accumulated pathogenic Qi. Releasing the area around the navel will help to release both physical and emotional traumas. The suggested method is as follows:

- Apply Ji dian fa and Zhen fa to the area all around the navel.
- Imagine eight doorways around Ren8, all 0.5 cun away. Think of them as representing the eight directions of a compass. Starting from the east at the doorway that corresponds to KD16 on the right, work around these points using An fa and Rou fa. Work with your patient's breath, applying pressure with their exhalation to take you to the Ying Qi level, maintain the pressure at that level and apply anti-clockwise Rou fa, gradually kneading up to the Wei Qi level at the surface. Your intention is to draw the pathogenic Qi up and out of the body through the navel. Apply this method three times, dispersing with Zhen fa, Ji dian fa and Pai fa in between. The third time when you have pressed down into the Ying Qi level, maintain the pressure and stretch the underlying tissue slightly by pushing your thumb away from the navel. Ask your patient to breathe into the pressure then, as before, use anti-clockwise Rou fa to draw up to the Wei Qi level.

Working under the ribs

To help release the diaphragm, move stagnation in the Middle Jiao, and improve the functions of the lungs, liver, gallbladder, stomach and spleen, the suggested method is as follows:

- Work under the ribs, moving gradually from the area of Liv13 on the right to Liv13 on the left using An fa and Rou fa with both thumbs. Work with your patient's breath, applying pressure with their exhala-

tion. To provide deeper stimulation, ask your patient to breathe deeply into your pressure a few times.

General tips for treating digestive problems

- Work on the back first, the Governing Vessel, Bladder channel, sacrum and hips, any relevant Back Shu points, Governing Vessel or Huatuojiaji points.
- Work distally on the appropriate leg, and sometimes the arm channels, stimulating your chosen distal points as you work.
- Work the chest and ribs to soothe and disperse Qi using the basis of the area foundation routine.
- Work the abdomen last.
- Use the simple abdominal routine as a basis for your local work.
- If on palpation of the abdomen you found knots, adhesion and accumulation, consider using some of the abdominal release work.

To help you plan a Tui na treatment for digestive ailments, see Table 12.1 for some suggestions of useful techniques to consider including in the treatment of common patterns of disharmony.

Case studies

To help illustrate the treatment of digestive ailments, three cases of patients I have treated follow.

Excessive belching and hypochondrial pain

Main complaint

Avi, a 38-year-old actor, had been suffering with what he described as excessive belching for the previous 18 months. He said he wanted to belch all the time, but he could usually control it if he was in public. When he was alone he was belching almost constantly. Recently it had become worse and he was starting to notice it when he was on stage. It was making him really angry. He told me straight away that he did not really believe in complementary medicine but the doctor could not find anything wrong with him and a friend had recommended me so he thought he would try it for a few sessions to see if it made any difference.

The belching was very loud and worse after eating. He had a distending pain under his ribs that came and went and was worse when he was stressed.

Secondary complaints

He had an oppressive feeling in his chest and found himself sighing and yawning frequently to ease the sensation. He also had a feeling of restriction in his throat as if something was stuck there. Emotionally he was very frustrated both with his acting career and with his family.

Palpation and observation

Avi had a wiry build and he looked tense. On palpation, the area under his ribs was Full and tender on pressure and there was tenderness at Liv14. The area around his navel was congested and knotted.

Table 12.1 Suggestions for the treatment of digestive ailments

Presenting disharmony	Useful treatment techniques
Spleen-Qi Xu Spleen- and Kidney-Yang Xu	Lifting–grasping from the sacrum to the nape about 10 times Palm Ya fa plus Rou fa up the spine and over points on the abdomen Clockwise palm and forearm Rou fa over Back Shu points and Front Mu points Clockwise Mo fa along Yin channels of the legs Tai chi Mo fa on the abdomen Ca fa along the Bladder channel of the back and across Back Shu points Ca fa at KD1, Du14 and Du4 for Yang Xu Palm Zhen fa over points on the abdomen and back Direct and indirect moxa of points
Liver-Qi stagnation Qi stagnation in the intestines	Pinching–grasping and kneading–grasping along the leg channels Gun fa on the back, hips and the sacrum area Rou fa hips and the sacrum Tan bo fa over the Bladder channel Back Shu points Ya fa at GB30 Tui fa, Zhen fa and Ji dian fa to the chest Lifting–grasping the abdomen Striking techniques on the back and limbs Cuo fa to the ribs Abdominal release work Cupping on the back and abdomen Gua sha on the back channels
Accumulation of Damp	Pai fa and joined palm Ji fa to the limbs and back Pai fa to the abdomen Pinching–grasping leg Yin channels Dredging Tui fa along the leg channels Indirect moxa over the abdominal area and points
Accumulation of Cold	Ca fa along the spine towards the head Zhen fa on the abdomen Gun fa along the back Warming palm Direct and indirect moxa of points
Accumulation of Heat	Ca fa along the spine towards the coccyx Gua sha or Gua fa down the Governing Vessel and along the Bladder channel of the back Nipping–grasping along the spine
Blood/Yin Xu	Tai chi Mo fa on the abdomen Mo fa along the Yin channels of the legs Palm Rou fa to the abdominal points Figure-of-eight Tui fa around the relevant Back Shu points, i.e. BL17 Warming palm to the abdomen

Tongue

His tongue was normal.

Pulse

His pulse was Wiry.

Diagnosis

The diagnosis was stagnation of Liver-Qi invading the Stomach.

Treatment principle

This was to disperse stagnant Qi, soothe the Liver and descend rebellious Stomach-Qi.

Treatment

With the patient lying prone

- Tui fa and Rou fa along the Bladder channel from the nape to the sacrum

- Compound technique pinching–grasping along the Bladder channel from the nape to the sacrum three times on each side
- Double-handed Gun fa along the Bladder channel to the level of the waist
- Tan bo fa over the paraspinal muscles from BL17 to BL21
- Yi zhi chan tui fa to stimulate BL17, BL18 and BL19
- Three-finger Ji dian fa from BL17 to BL21 using medium rhythmic striking
- Ya fa plus Rou fa to stimulate GB30
- Tui fa to dredge the Gallbladder channel

With the patient supine

- Yi zhi chan tui fa to stimulate Liv3, GB34, SJ6 and PC6
- Pinching–grasping, kneading–grasping, nipping–grasping, loose-fist Pai fa and five-finger Ji dian fa to the Liver and Gallbladder channels in his legs and

the San Jiao and Pericardium channels in his arms to move Qi and dissipate stagnation
- Tui fa, Ji dian fa and Zhen fa to his chest
- Compound technique, pushing–pressing in the axilla and the subclavicular fossa
- Compound technique, kneading–grasping to his pectoral muscles
- An fa to stimulate ST12
- Tui fa and Rou fa to his ribs
- Yi zhi chan tui fa to stimulate Liv14 and Ren12
- Palm Zhen fa over Liv14 and Ren12
- Tui fa, forearm Rou fa and Mo fa to his abdomen
- Compound technique, lifting–grasping over his ribs and to his abdomen
- Ji dian fa around his navel
- Whisking–sweeping and Ca fa to his ribs

Advice to the patient

I suggested to Avi that he reduce his coffee intake. He was drinking six strong cups a day. He was not getting enough exercise as far as he was concerned; he used to enjoy running but had got out of the habit. I encouraged him to take up running again as I thought it would help to move his Qi.

Progress and subsequent treatment

I gave Avi a total of six weekly treatments. After three treatments, things began to change. The plum stone throat and oppressive feeling in his chest were the first symptoms to be alleviated. He was encouraged by the changes that he felt and said he thought that Tui na was doing him some good and would continue with this form of treatment. Over the 6 weeks I worked with the above treatment and added more abdominal release work under his ribs and around his navel, getting him involved by working with his breath. His belching and hypochondrial discomfort diminished each week. He relaxed and communicated more with each treatment. He was running again, and he was also meditating for 10 minutes every day (he had given this up a few years ago). When he came in for his sixth treatment, he sat back in the chair, smiled at me and told me that the treatment had worked. He had not belched all week and had no discomfort. He looked very different from the man I had met a few weeks before.

Constipation

Main complaint

Laura, aged 43, was suffering with constipation and tiredness. She felt bloated and uncomfortable in her abdomen most of the time. Her stools were hard, dry and infrequent (about twice a week). The previous few years had been very stressful; she had had two miscarriages over this time. She was very tired, especially in the morning and around her period. I distinctly got the impression that she was holding on to a lot of emotion and had become accustomed to being 'very nice' in order to protect herself.

Secondary complaints

She had temporal and vertical headaches, especially premenstrually and during her period which was regular but had become very light over the past year. She had floaters most of the time, dizziness when she was hungry and on the first day of her period, and dry skin. She had also been having a lot of lower backache for the previous 12 months and had been seeing an osteopath for treatment of this. She urinated frequently (every hour) during the day. Generally she felt cold easily and her hands were cold.

Palpation and observation

There was general tenderness in the lower left side of her abdomen and at Liv13 and ST25. There were several areas of knotting in her lower abdomen.

Tongue

Her tongue was pale and dry.

Pulse

Her pulse was Choppy.

Diagnosis

The diagnosis was Blood Xu leading to dryness and stagnation of Qi in the Intestines. Her Kidney-Yang was also Deficient.

Treatment principle

This was to disperse stagnation and encourage the movement of Qi in the Intestines, nourish Blood and warm Kidney-Yang.

Treatment

With the patient lying prone

- Tui fa along the Bladder channel from the nape to the sacrum gently and until warm
- Forearm Rou fa over BL14, BL17, BL20 and BL23
- Gun fa from BL23 to BL25
- Ca fa across the lower back

With the patient supine

- Tui fa and Mo fa slowly and gently along the Yin channels of the legs following the flow of the primary meridians
- An fa and clockwise Rou fa slowly and gently to stimulate Liv3, Liv8, SP6 and ST36 focusing on pushing into the Ying Qi level
- Tui fa across her chest and ribs
- An fa and Rou fa in the intercostal spaces
- Mo fa over her lower ribs focusing on Liv13
- Tui fa, tai chi Mo fa and palm Rou fa to her abdomen for 10 minutes, focusing on Ren12, ST25 and Ren4 with clockwise palm Rou fa
- Zhen fa over Ren4
- Cat's paw across her abdomen

Ancillary therapies

Direct moxa was used in the form of three small cones on BL17, BL19, BL20, BL23 and Ren4.

Advice to the patient

I showed Laura how to breathe into her belly and how to apply some simple self-massage to her abdomen.

Progress and subsequent treatments

Over the next few treatments I began to introduce some of the abdominal release work to clear the knotted areas that I had found. This proved to be very effective. (This work keeps the patient working with you; as you encourage them to breathe into areas of accumulated Qi, their awareness and breath begin to release what has been held.) Memories and emotion surfaced as we worked together over the next few weeks and her bowel movements started to come more frequently, her energy levels started to rise and her backache was much improved. I worked with Laura weekly for 12 weeks. In the second half of her menstrual cycle I continued with release work on her abdomen and some deeper work in her sacrum and hips with Ya fa and Rou fa, encouraging Qi to move. During her period I worked more on her back and distally and very simply on her belly with Mo fa, Zhen fa and warming palm. In the postmenstrual week, I worked very gently with the treatment described above without any release work.

Gradually I showed Laura more abdominal work that she could do herself between treatments; this makes a huge difference when you are limited to treatments once a week or less.

By the end of the 12 weeks, Laura had gone through quite a transformation. She was having regular daily bowel movements that were normal in shape and no longer dry, she had no backache or headaches and she felt generally warmer. She said her energy was back to how it was before she had her children; she felt positive in herself and had started playing the cello again which she had not touched for over 7 years. I still see Laura once a month for maintenance treatment.

Diarrhea

Main complaint

David, aged 46, had been suffering with diarrhea for the previous 5 years. His stools were very loose, watery and urgent. The diarrhea started from the time he woke up in the morning and was accompanied by some abdominal pain; it lasted until about midday after which he was okay. On average, he would have to go to the toilet six or seven times every morning. Getting to work on the train was becoming a nightmare; he knew every toilet en route and had to stop at least twice on the way. He was very stressed and anxious about it. His appetite was up and down and he often felt bloated. He had stopped eating breakfast in case it made his morning diarrhea worse. He craved sweet things and ate pasta several times a week but generally his diet was quite good.

He had been made redundant from a job that he loved 6 years before and was dissatisfied and unfulfilled in his current work. He was constantly worrying and trying to work out what he should do.

Secondary complaints

David felt easily tired. He had lower backache from time to time. Other than that he was in good health.

Palpation and observation

His abdomen was cold to the touch. Ren12 and Ren6 felt very Empty on pressure.

Tongue

His tongue was pale with scallops and with a thin white coating.

Pulse

His pulse was Weak and Deep.

Diagnosis

The diagnosis was Spleen- and Kidney-Yang Xu.

Treatment principle

This was to warm and strengthen Kidney- and Spleen-Yang, stop the diarrhea and calm the mind.

Treatment

With the patient lying prone

Using red flower balm I applied:

- Tui fa along the Governing Vessel from Du2 to Du14 until warm
- Palm Ya fa up the Governing Vessel followed by clockwise palm Rou fa
- Tui fa and palm Rou fa along the Bladder channel from the nape to the sacrum
- Compound technique, pinching–grasping along the Bladder channel from the nape to the sacrum three times on each side
- Gun fa along the Bladder channel, concentrating on the areas of BL20 and BL23 until they were very warm. I coordinated this with An fa and Tui fa down the backs of his legs along the Bladder channel
- Yi zhi chan tui fa on BL20, BL23 and BL25, followed by forearm Rou fa
- Compound technique, lifting–grasping along the Governing Vessel from Du2 to Du14 ten times
- Ca fa across Du4 and Du14
- Ca fa to KD1

With the patient supine

- Tui fa and Rou fa on his legs, working down the Stomach and up the Spleen channels until warm. An fa to stimulate KD3 and SP6 focusing on pushing Qi up the channels into the Kidney and Spleen
- Ca fa along the Yin channels of the legs until hot
- Yi zhi chan tui fa on ST36
- Tai chi Mo fa to his abdomen in an anti-clockwise direction for 5 minutes
- Forearm Rou fa clockwise over Ren12, ST25 and Ren6 plus Gun fa down his legs along the Stomach channel

- Palm An fa and Rou fa over Ren12, ST25, Ren8 and Ren6. At the same time I applied An fa to Du20 with my left thumb
- Palm Zhen fa over the above points

To finish

I applied warming palm with one palm over Ren8 and the other over his forehead with the intention of calming his Shen.

Ancillary therapies

I used moxa on ginger at Du4, BL23, BL20 and Ren12, and moxa on salt at Ren8, with three substantial cones on each point.

Advice to the patient

I advised David to drink some ginger tea in the morning to warm his Stomach- and Spleen-Qi and encouraged him to start eating breakfast again. I suggested that he ate more short grain organic brown rice and less pasta. I also showed him how to apply moxa with a moxa stick to KD3 and Ren12 and suggested that he did this every day between treatments as he could only come weekly.

Progress and subsequent treatments

I continued to treat David weekly as described above for 10 weeks, often finishing treatment with warming palm over his head, eyes, abdomen or lower back and some gentle work on his face and head to calm his Shen. David continued to use moxa between treatments and I showed him how to apply some simple massage to his abdomen and lower back and some Qigong exercises to help to strengthen his Spleen- and Kidney-Qi. After 5 weeks David had noticed some significant improvements. He was going to the toilet three times in the morning and his stools, although still loose, were no longer watery and were less urgent. He was feeling generally more in control. After 10 weeks, he was passing soft but formed stools twice a day, once in the morning and once after lunch without any urgency; he had no abdominal bloating or discomfort. He was no longer tired and said he was beginning to feel quite stable in himself. His tongue was less pale and the scallops almost entirely gone. His pulse was stronger. I gave him two treatments a fortnight apart and then three monthly treatments to maintain and further the progress. He now comes for treatment about twice a year, just for an 'MOT' as he calls it.

CHAPTER **13**

Gynecological problems

Tui na is an effective form of treatment for a variety of gynecological problems. It is especially useful in the treatment of menstrual disorders such as dysmenorrhea, irregular periods, amenorrhea, fibroids and premenstrual tension (PMT). It is also of great benefit in the treatment of infertility and for menopausal ailments, both of which have become increasingly common reasons for women to seek out treatment with oriental medicine.

Tui na treatment of gynecological problems has two main areas of focus:

1. Treating the presenting disharmony such as stagnation or Cold in the Uterus
2. Releasing and clearing congestion, accumulation and knotted or hypertense fascia

There are several key factors involved in creating a woman's fertility and healthy menstrual cycle:

- An abundant supply of blood
- The smooth and harmonious movement of Qi and Blood through the Chong Mai, Ren Mai and Uterus
- A warm Uterus
- The strength and balance of Kidney-Yin and Kidney-Yang
- An abdomen free of congestion, knotting and accumulation

Depending on the underlying disharmony and upon what you find when palpating the abdomen, treatment generally involves a combination of tonifying and nourishing Qi and Blood, dispersing Qi and Blood stasis, regulating the flow of Qi and Blood through the Chong and Ren Mai, warming the Uterus, warming and strengthening Kidney-Yang, nourishing Kidney-Yin, clearing and dredging obstructing pathogenic factors, releasing the abdomen and improving the alignment of the fallopian tubes and ovaries.

Abdominal release work

It is hugely important to keep the abdomen free of congestion so that Qi and Blood can flow freely and harmoniously through the Uterus. Accumulation and stagnation of Qi, Blood and pathogenic factors can lead to problems such as ovarian cysts, endometriosis, fibroids, PMT and infertility. Stagnation is a major factor in gynecological conditions; this can be caused by a deficiency such as Qi and Blood Xu or Kidney-Yang Xu or by retention and accumulation of pathogenic factors such as Cold, Damp and Phlegm.

Abdominal release work enables Qi and Blood to move and helps to disperse accumulations, adhesions and knotting. The uterus is attached within the abdomen by tendons, which can become tight and tense. This is often due to accumulation of stagnant Qi in the intestines, commonly caused by emotional stress. This tension and stagnation in the fascia of the abdomen can cause the fallopian tubes to twist and the ovaries to become out of alignment, which can interfere with ovulation and increase the tendency to develop problems such as ovarian cysts.

Applying the abdominal release work described on pages 151–152 is, in my experience, of great benefit in the treatment of gynecological problems. In addition to this, I have found the following methods to be effective for clearing stagnation in the Uterus, helping to balance the ebb and flow of Yin and Yang throughout the monthly cycle, for aiding ovulation and encouraging the correct alignment of the fallopian tubes and ovaries:

- Kneading–grasping compound technique applied to the lower abdomen using both hands, with your fingers to one side of the uterus and your thumbs at the other. Work deeply into tight and congested areas.
- With your patient lying with her knees up, apply An fa in a rocking, wave-like motion similar to the cat's paw technique, using the ulnar edge of your hand horizontally across Ren2 and ST30. Rock from one side to the other about 100 times.
- With your patient lying supine again, apply palm Rou fa to Ren4 for a minimum of 5 minutes.
- Apply warming palm to the abdomen with your attention at the level of the Uterus. Work with Sun Qi if there is Yang Xu or Cold, and Moon Qi if there is Blood or Yin Deficiency.

General tips for treating gynecological problems

- In the second half of the cycle, work more dynamically, focusing on moving and invigorating Qi and Blood, dispersing stasis, and clearing and dredging pathogenic factors.
- In the first half of the cycle, work more gently with a Yin approach, focusing on nourishing and tonifying Deficiency.

- In the case of menorrhagia, local abdominal work and release work should only be performed in the postmenstrual week.
- Work on the patient's back, hips and sacrum first, stimulating relevant points, areas and channels according to your diagnosis. Stimulation of the 8 liao points from BL31 to BL34, and generally the area of the sacrum, ilium, iliopsoas and gluteus, with Rou fa, Gun fa and Ya fa is very effective for moving stagnation and warming the Uterus.
- Work distally on appropriate channels and points.
- Work on the chest and ribs if the patient has signs of Qi stagnating in the chest or has emotional symptoms such as depression and irritability or insomnia.
- Apply local abdominal work after you have worked on the back, distally and on the chest.
- Use the abdominal release work if there are areas of knotting, congestion and adhesion or stagnation and accumulation of pathogenic factors.
- Work on the face and head to finish if the patient has emotional symptoms, headaches or insomnia.

To help you plan a Tui na treatment for gynecological problems, see Table 13.1 for some suggestions of techniques to consider including in the treatment of common patterns of disharmony. In all cases the foundation area routine for the abdomen can be used as an outline for the local work, with the addition of any abdominal release work and techniques and methods relevant to the presenting disharmony.

Table 13.1 Suggestions for the treatment of gynecological problems

Presenting disharmony	Useful treatment techniques
Stagnation of Qi and Blood stasis	Tan bo fa along the paraspinal muscles, focusing on relevant Back Shu points, i.e. BL17, BL18, BL23 and the 8 liao (BL31–BL34) Ji dian fa, Ji fa and Pai fa along the Bladder and Gallbladder channels Pinching–grasping along the Bladder channel Pinching–grasping and kneading–pinching along the medial aspect of the leg along the Spleen and Liver channels Gun fa, Rou fa and Na fa to the lower back, sacrum and hips Ya fa plus Rou fa to GB30 Chest and hypochondrium routine emphasizing Ji dian fa and Zhen fa Palm Ya fa to SP12, hold for 2 minutes then release Gun fa and Zhen fa to the abdomen Gua sha on the back along the Governing Vessel and Bladder channel Medium cupping over the sacrum, hips and lower back
Accumulation and stagnation of Damp Cold	Palm Rou fa along the Governing Vessel from the coccyx to nape Gua fa on the back along the Governing Vessel and Bladder channel Coordinated Gun fa and forearm Rou fa to the Bladder channel along the back and back of the leg Tan bo fa along the Bladder channel from the nape to the sacrum Thumb and forearm Rou fa, Ca fa and Zhen fa to the 8 liao Ca fa along the Governing Vessel from Du2 to Du14 and along the Bladder channel from the nape to the buttocks Pai fa and joined palm Ji fa to the back, hips and legs Ya fa to GB30 until very warm Tui fa and Ca fa to the abdomen along the Ren, Stomach and Spleen channels Ca fa across SP12 Forearm Rou fa across Ren8 and ST25 Zhen fa, Gun fa and hollow palm Pai fa to the abdomen Ya fa to Ren6 until very warm Moxa on salt at Ren8 Moxa on ginger at Ren6, Ren12, Du4 Indirect moxa over the sacrum and lower abdomen or moxa box over the sacrum

Table 13.1 Suggestions for the treatment of gynecological problems—cont'd

Presenting disharmony	Useful treatment techniques
Accumulation and stagnation of Damp Heat	Gua fa on the back along the Governing Vessel and Bladder channel Nipping–grasping along the Governing Vessel from Du14 to Du2 Ca fa to Du14 Nipping and kneading and Ji dian fa to relevant points Pinching–grasping and nipping–grasping to Yin and Yang channels of the arms and legs Pai fa, Ji fa and Ji dian fa to the back, hips, sacrum, arms and legs Chest and hypochondrium routine with emphasis on pushing–pressing the supraclavicular fossa, Zhen fa and Ji dian fa Lifting and grasping, Zhen fa and Pai fa to the abdomen Gua sha along the Governing Vessel and Bladder channel Cupping to the lower back, sacrum and hips
Qi and Blood Xu Spleen-Qi Xu	Forearm, palm and thumb Rou fa to the Back Shu points BL17, BL19, BL20 and BL23 Palm Mo fa over the Spleen, Liver and Kidney Back Shu points Lifting and grasping along the spine from Du2 to Du14 Gun fa and Ca fa to the lower back and sacrum Tui fa, Mo fa and Rou fa along the Yin channels of the legs Mo fa over Ren12 coordinated with Tui fa down the leg along the Stomach channel Tai chi Mo fa and Zhen fa on the abdomen Holding relevant points and directing Qi and intention Warming palm to the abdomen and spleen Direct moxa with rice grain cones to points
Liver- and Kidney-Yin Xu Kidney-Yin Xu	Tui fa down the back along the Bladder channel Forearm or palm Rou fa to BL23, BL52, BL18 and the 8 liao Figure-of-eight Tui fa around the Kidney and Liver Back Shu points Gun fa to the lower back Ca fa to KD1 Tui fa, Mo fa, An fa and Rou fa to the lower leg along the Liver and Kidney channels Tui fa and Mo fa to the ribs and abdomen Palm Rou fa and tai chi Mo fa over Ren4 Zhen fa to the abdomen Holding relevant points and directing Qi and intention Warming palm to the Kidneys and Liver drawing in Moon Qi
Kidney-Yang Xu Stagnation of Cold	Tui fa, palm Ya fa and Rou fa along the Governing Vessel from Du2 to Du14 Lifting–grasping up the spine from Du2 to Du14 Coordinated Gun fa and forearm Rou fa to the lower back, sacrum and down the legs along the Bladder channel Ca fa along the Governing Vessel, across Du4, BL23 and BL52 and the 8 liao (BL31–BL34) Figure-of-eight Tui fa around the kidneys and warming palm drawing in Sun Qi Palm Ya fa and Ca fa at the inguinal area across SP12 and along the inner medial thigh Rou fa, Gun fa and kneading–grasping along the Yin channels of the leg Palm and forearm Rou fa over Ren12, Ren8 and Ren4 Tui fa and Ca fa along the Ren Mai and Kidney channels in the abdomen from the top of the pubic bone to the navel Zhen fa over Ren8 and other chosen abdominal points Thumb Rou fa to Du20 Moxa on ginger at Du4, BL23, Ren6 Moxa on salt at Ren8; moxa stick over abdomen and sacrum or moxa box Direct rice grain cones to distal points
Blood-Heat Empty Heat in the Blood	Gua fa, pinching–grasping and nipping–grasping to the back along the Governing Vessel and Bladder channel Nipping–grasping and Ca fa to Du14 Thumb Rou fa and kneading–pinching to BL14, BL15, BL17 and BL19 Gun fa to the lower back, hips and sacrum Kneading–grasping, pinching–grasping and nipping–grasping along the Yin channels of the legs Pushing and pressing the supraclavicular fossa, axilla and popliteal fossa An fa and Rou fa to the chest Tui fa and whisking–sweeping to the ribs Forearm Rou fa to the abdomen Kneading–nipping PC8 Ca fa at KD1 Gua sha on the back along the Governing Vessel and Bladder channel Medium or empty cupping along the Bladder channel

Case studies

To help illustrate the treatment of gynecological problems, three cases of patients I have treated follow.

Dysmenorrhea

Main complaint

Karen, aged 30, came for treatment to help with her period pains and premenstrual tension. She had suffered with intense period pains for the previous 4 years and often had to take time off work because she felt so awful. She had pain every month on the first day of her period and every few months it was particularly intense. On these occasions the pain was often accompanied by nausea, sometimes with vomiting and diarrhea; she felt light-headed, and very drained but also restless. She applied a hot water bottle to her abdomen and after an hour or so she was able to lie down and rub her abdomen and would eventually fall asleep. When she woke the pain was much better but she felt very tired and could not do much for the rest of the day. The flow started hesitantly with pinkish blood, which turned dark by the end of the first day; there were substantial dark red clots. She had a regular 29–30 day cycle. The bleed lasted for 7 days; the last 2 days the flow was very light and brown. She now always took painkillers on the first day of her period, which she thought helped to take the edge off the pain.

Premenstrually, Karen felt irritable or depressed and weepy, her breasts were sore and distended and her abdomen felt uncomfortable and bloated.

Secondary complaint

Karen also had frequent headaches around her eyes and temples that were worse in the premenstrual week. She felt very stiff in her neck and the tops of her shoulders.

Palpation and observation

When I saw Karen, it was day 21 of her cycle. Her abdomen looked and felt generally distended. There were several areas of knotting and congestion in the small intestine below her navel and the area under her ribs was very tight and tender on pressure, especially on the right.

Tongue

Her tongue had a purple hue and was red at the tip, with some scallops at the sides, and distended and purple sublingual veins.

Pulse

Her pulse was Deep and Wiry.

Diagnosis

The diagnosis was stagnation of Qi and Blood, accumulation and congestion in the abdomen, rebellious Liver-Qi, underlying Qi and Blood Xu.

Treatment principle

In the second half of her cycle, treatment was to move Qi and Blood, eliminate stasis, disperse accumulation and congestion in the abdomen and soothe and regulate the Liver. In the first half of her cycle, it was to invigorate Qi, nourish Blood, soothe the Liver and strengthen the Spleen.

Treatment

Second half of cycle treatment

With the patient lying prone
- Tui fa on the back down the Bladder channel
- Kneading–grasping GB21 on one side and heel of palm Rou fa down the Bladder channel on the other side; repeat on the other side
- Tan bo fa along the paraspinal muscles focusing on BL17, BL18, BL23 and the 8 liao (BL31–BL34)
- Gun fa over the lower back, sacrum and buttocks accompanied by Rou fa, Na fa and An fa down the back of the legs
- Gun fa down the back of the legs plus forearm Rou fa over the lower back, sacrum and buttocks
- Pushing–pressing BL40
- Ya fa to BL53, BL36 and GB30
- Heel of palm Rou fa to the sacrum
- Ca fa over the lower back and sacrum with wood-lock oil

With the patient supine
- Yi zhi chan tui fa to stimulate SP4 on the right, PC6 on the left, Liv3 on the left and LI4 on the right
- Palm Ya fa to SP12
- Kneading–grasping and kneading–pinching down the Spleen and Liver channels stimulating SP10 and SP8 on the way
- The basis of the chest and ribs routine with an emphasis on Tui fa, Ji dian fa, Zhen fa and pushing–pressing

Local abdominal work I used the abdominal foundation routine as the basis for the local work, integrating the abdominal release work to break up the congested areas in her lower abdomen and under her ribs, as follows:
- An fa and Rou fa to stimulate ST25, ST29 and Ren4
- Kneading–grasping the lower abdomen with both hands
- Palm Rou fa and Zhen fa over Ren4

Finally I did 5 minutes' work on her face using Tui fa, Ma fa, Rou fa and warming palm.

First half of cycle treatment

With the patient lying prone
- Tui fa and Rou fa on the back along the Bladder channel
- Forearm Rou fa over BL17, BL18, BL20, BL23 and the 8 liao
- Gun fa over the lower back, sacrum and buttocks coordinated with Tui fa, Rou fa and An fa down the backs of the legs along the Bladder channel
- Ca fa either side of the spine and across the sacrum

With the patient supine
- Tui fa, Mo fa and Rou fa along the Spleen and Liver channels
- Holding and connecting with my middle fingers SP6 and SP12

Local abdominal work

- Mo fa over Ren12 coordinated with Tui fa down the leg along the Stomach channel
- Holding and connecting ST36 and ST30
- Tai chi Mo fa on the lower abdomen
- Zhen fa and palm Rou fa to Ren4
- Warming palm over the Uterus and Spleen and Liver

Finally I applied the foundation routine for the head and face.

Advice to the patient

Karen worked at a computer all day so I advised her to increase her exercise and to do more exercise in the second half of her cycle to encourage Qi and Blood to move. I encouraged her to join a yoga class, showed her how to massage her abdomen and suggested she do this every day.

Progress and subsequent treatments

Karen came for treatment once a week for the next 3 months. We continued with treatment as described above and made steady progress; the pain became less intense, the blood flow less hesitant and scanty at the start and her premenstrual symptoms were diminishing. When she came for treatment after the third period, she reported a marked difference. She said it took her a bit by surprise because she did not have any mood changes or sore breasts. She described the pain as more of a background, dragging sensation without any of the previous intensity and the blood was generally less dark and clotty. She had not experienced any of the rebellious Qi symptoms and had noticed that she had not been having her usual headaches.

I continued to treat Karen on a fortnightly basis for another three cycles, timing the treatments to coincide with her pre- and postmenstrual weeks. I continue to see her on a monthly basis in her premenstrual week for maintenance treatments. She no longer has anything more than a mild ache on the first day of her period and she has had no further problems with PMT.

Fertility

Main complaint

Danielle, aged 42, worked in the media world and had a very lively and exciting lifestyle involving long hours, both working and socializing. She did not have any children and it was only over the previous few years that she realized that she would like to have a child. She had become pregnant 3 years before but had miscarried at 10 weeks. Since then she had tried two cycles of in vitro fertilization (IVF) which had proved unsuccessful at the stage of implantation. An ultrasound scan had revealed a small cyst on her left ovary; her hormone levels were within the normal range. She was planning to start another IVF cycle in a month's time.

In the past her periods had always been regular and painless but over the previous few years her cycle had become longer, around 31 days, and she was experiencing intense pains in her abdomen and sacral area on the first 2 days of her period. The blood was bright red with a lot of purplish clots; the flow was light and lasted for 5 days. She used a hot water bottle to ease the pain which she described as intense. She felt cold easily.

Secondary complaints

Danielle had lower backache, which she felt around her sacrum and iliac crest. She urinated frequently and always had to get up once at night. Other than that she said she felt very well and her energy levels were good.

Palpation and observation

Danielle's abdomen was distinctly cold to the touch; she was aware of this herself and told me she often tried to warm it up with a hot water bottle. On palpation there was discomfort around the area of ST30 on the left-hand side; the area around Ren4 was noticeably hollow to look at and very empty on pressure. There were several areas of congestion in her lower abdomen. Her navel was being pulled slightly diagonally in the direction of her left hip.

Tongue

Her tongue was pale.

Pulse

Her pulse was Deep, Slow and Weak.

Diagnosis

The diagnosis was Kidney-Yang Xu, and stagnation of Cold obstructing the Uterus.

Treatment principle

This was to warm Kidney-Yang, disperse Cold and accumulated congestion, warm the Uterus, and encourage Qi and Blood to move harmoniously through the Uterus.

Treatment

With the patient lying prone

- Tui fa and palm Rou fa along the Bladder channel from the nape to the sacrum and along the Governing Vessel from Du2 to Du14
- Double-handed Gun fa along the Bladder channel from the shoulders to the waist
- Coordinated Gun fa and Tui fa. Gun fa in the lower back especially around BL23 and Tui fa from the buttocks down the legs along the Bladder channel
- Coordinated Gun fa and forearm Rou fa. Forearm Rou fa over BL23, the sacrum and 8 liao (BL31–BL34) and the ileum and Gun fa down the legs along the Bladder channel
- Clockwise thumb Rou fa to stimulate Du4, Du14 and Du20
- Yi zhi chan tui fa to stimulate BL23 and BL31
- Rou fa either side of the sacrum with fingers interlaced, using the heels of the palms
- Elbow Ya fa plus Rou fa to GB30 and BL54
- Lifting–grasping along the Governing Vessel from Du2 to Du14
- Ca fa across Du4, BL23 and BL52, across the sacrum and either side of the spine along the Bladder channel using red flower oil

With the patient supine

- Tui fa, Rou fa and kneading–grasping along the Yin channels of the legs, following the flow of the primary meridians
- Clockwise thumb Rou fa to stimulate KD3 and KD7
- Ca fa along the medial thigh over the three Yin channels
- Ca fa on the thigh along the Stomach channel
- Single-finger Ji dian fa to stimulate ST36
- Palm Ya fa and Ca fa to the inguinal area over SP12

Local abdominal work

- Palm Tui fa from Ren2 to Ren15 and along the Stomach channel from ST21 to ST30
- Tai chi Mo fa focusing on Ren6 and Ren4
- Abdominal release work to break up areas of congestion
- Kneading–grasping the lower abdomen with both hands, working deeply into tight and congested areas
- With her knees up, I applied An fa in a rocking, wave-like motion across Ren2 and ST30 with the ulnar edge of my hand
- Palm Rou fa and Zhen fa to Ren4 for several minutes
- Warming palm to the Uterus and Kidneys using breath and intention to project Sun Qi

Ancillary therapies

I applied three small moxa cones directly to Du4, Du14, BL23 and BL31 after applying the work on her back. I applied three large moxa cones on salt to Ren8 and three large cones directly to Ren4, blowing the smoke as they burned to help disperse the Cold before I applied the local abdominal work.

Advice to the patient

I showed Danielle how to apply moxa with a moxa stick to her abdomen and to KD3 and advised her to apply this every day for 10 minutes on her abdomen and for 3 minutes on each of the Kidney points. I also advised her to eat warm foods and to stay off the salads and icy drinks that she was fond of.

Progress and subsequent treatments

As Danielle wanted to start IVF within a month, she came for treatment three times a week for the next 3 weeks so that we could concentrate on clearing the congestion and warming her Uterus and Kidney-Yang. She continued to use moxa between treatments. I also showed her how to apply some self-massage to her abdomen, lower back and thighs. By the time she started her IVF cycle, her abdomen was feeling quite warm and the areas of congestion and tenderness had dispersed; she also had no more discomfort in her lower back.

During the IVF cycle I continued to treat Danielle once a week up to the point of egg collection. I no longer applied abdominal release work but instead focused on warming the Uterus and stimulating the ovaries. The work on the back and the distal work remained the same as that described above. The local work consisted of Tui fa, tai chi Mo fa, palm Rou fa and Zhen fa plus wave-like An fa over Ren2 and ST30 and Zhen fa to stimulate the extra point Zi gong. The application of moxa remained the same.

Egg collection was successful. I treated her twice more before implantation and once immediately after implantation. This treatment simply consisted of moxa on BL23 and Du4 followed by gentle holding An fa applied to the points with my middle fingers for several minutes and warming palm over the kidneys and sacrum. I applied three small moxa cones to SP6 followed by holding An fa and finally warming palm to the Uterus for 10 minutes.

I am happy to say that at the time of writing this book, Danielle was 19 weeks pregnant.

Menopause

Main complaint

Brenda, aged 52, was recommended by a friend to come for treatment to help her through the menopause. Her periods had become increasingly irregular over the previous 2 years and her last period was over 5 months before. She was particularly bothered by hot flushes and sweating which had become worse over the previous 6 months and which had begun to disturb her sleep. She woke several times during the night drenched in sweat with her heart racing. She frequently had palpitations when she lay down to go to sleep. She felt tired all the time and was easily stressed, irritable and anxious. She was worried about her sleep, as she had suffered with insomnia in the past.

Secondary complaints

She had lower backache, and irritable bowel syndrome (IBS) which was worse with stress and when she ate too many sweet things, which she craved all the time. She had dry skin and vaginal dryness which was also making her anxious.

Palpation and observation

Brenda had a malar flush. Her skin was dry to the touch. On palpation of her abdomen, the Ren Mai and Kidney channels felt very Empty, especially at Ren4, Ren12 and Ren14. There was marked tenderness at ST25, KD24 and KD27.

Tongue

Her tongue was red and dry, and it had lots of irregular cracks and no coating.

Pulse

Her pulse was Empty and Quick.

Diagnosis

The diagnosis was Kidney- and Heart-Yin Xu, Empty Heat in the Ren and Chong Mai.

Treatment principle

This was to nourish Yin, harmonize and tonify the Kidney and Heart, clear Empty Heat and soothe and calm the Shen.

Treatment

With the patient lying prone

- Tui fa and Rou fa along the course of the Bladder channel from the nape to the toes
- Gua Fa on the back along the Governing Vessel and Bladder channel
- Nipping–grasping along the Governing Vessel from Du14 to Du4
- Mo fa over BL14 and BL23 followed by holding the points with my middle fingers and focusing my attention on tonifying the Heart- and Kidney-Yin, visualizing Moon Qi moving through the points into the organs
- Figure-of-eight Tui fa around the Heart and Kidney Back Shu points

With the patient supine

- Holding SP4 on the right, PC6 on the left, then LU7 on the right and KD6 on the left with my middle fingers, intention focused on nourishing Kidney- and Heart-Yin and harmonizing the Ren and Chong Mai
- Tui fa, Mo fa and Rou fa along the Yin channels of the legs and arms
- Tui fa KD1
- Kneading–nipping KD2 and PC8
- Thumb Rou fa to stimulate SP6, KD9 and HT6

On the face

- Tui fa from Yintang to Du24
- Ma fa across the forehead
- Rou fa Yintang and Tai Yang
- Kneading–grasping the ears

On the chest

- Tui fa across the chest and from Ren22 to Ren17
- An fa, Rou fa and Ma fa across the intercostal spaces
- Kneading and grasping the pectoral muscles, stimulating HT1 and LU1

- Gentle Ji dian fa along the kidney channel from KD27 to KD25

On the abdomen

- Tui fa and tai chi Mo fa
- Palm Rou fa on Ren14 and Ren4
- Palm Zhen fa on Ren8 and Ren4
- Holding the uterus between both palms and projecting nourishing, cooling Moon Qi

Advice to the patient

I encouraged Brenda to see a colleague of mine who is a practitioner of natural nutrition to give her some support and advice with her diet. I taught her some simple self-massage to apply every day to her chest, abdomen and lower back and to KD1 and PC8.

Progress and subsequent treatments

Initially I saw Brenda weekly for 6 months. Over this time she went through a major transformation. She made significant changes to her diet and conquered her sugar addiction, started Qigong and tai chi classes and got a place at university to study anthropology. She responded very well to Tui na which she loved. Her sleep, energy and mood improved after three treatments and the sweating and flushes diminished gradually over the months. She has very few hot flushes now and those she has do not bother her. She now sees me every fortnight for maintenance and continued support.

The menopause is a time of great potential for women, a real rite of passage. I have witnessed some incredible transformations occur, from the stages of cleansing, grief and loss of what has been to the often awe-inspiring creation and birth of a new way of life. I have been fortunate enough to treat and support many women through this extremely challenging time and have personally found Tui na an invaluable form of treatment.

CHAPTER **14**

Headaches and hypertension

Headaches

Headaches are one of the most common symptoms that you will come across in practice. Some patients come for treatment with headaches as their main complaint, as is the case with migraine. They are frequently associated with a variety of ailments such as common colds, sinus problems, hay fever, digestive disorders and muscular skeletal problems.

Tui na is great for headaches; it can bring on-the-spot relief and, in the case of chronic headaches and migraine, regular treatments can produce excellent results.

There are many types of headache and the causes of these are wide and varied. A common 21st century cause is tension and stagnation of Qi in the Yang channel sinews due to stress, emotional holding patterns, excessive computer use and lack of appropriate exercise.

In the case of migraine which seems increasingly common, especially among women, there is a often a combination of stagnation and tension, usually in the Tai Yang and Shao Yang channel sinews, plus Deficiency of Blood and Yin and, consequently, rebellious Yang Qi rising.

In my practice I have found the most common headaches are those related to tension and stagnation of Qi in the Yang channel sinews of the neck, shoulders and back, digestive disharmonies leading to Qi stagnation and the production of Damp and Phlegm, Deficiency of Qi and Blood and Liver-Yang rising due to Deficient Liver-Blood or Liver/Kidney-Yin Xu.

Depending on your diagnosis of the underlying disharmony, Tui na treatment usually involves a combination of several elements, the most common being:

- Releasing the Yang channel sinews, expelling external pathogenic factors and moving and dispersing obstructed Wei Qi
- Strengthening and invigorating Qi and Blood and enabling clear Yang to rise
- Soothing Qi and soothing the Liver
- Nourishing Blood and Yin
- Tonifying the Kidneys
- Harmonizing the Middle Jiao and the Stomach and Intestines
- Tonifying the Spleen, dredging and eliminating Damp and Phlegm
- Descending rebellious Qi

General tips for treating headaches

- Take your time to palpate for tender local points and areas of holding and adhesion, particularly along the Tai Yang and Shao Yang channel sinews in the patient's neck, nape, shoulders and paraspinal muscles. Stimulate the most tender points with appropriate techniques and release the sinews as you come to work in the affected areas.
- At the beginning of treatment, do some work on the patient's head and face using the basis of the foundation routine for the head and face. Return to the local work at the end of the treatment.
- Release the neck, nape and shoulders and stimulate any relevant points in these areas.

- If necessary, do any work on the back next; for example, release stagnation and adhesion, stimulate relevant points such as Back Shu, Governing Vessel and Huatuojiaji points, and apply any nourishing Yin style work on the back such as tonifying the Kidneys.
- Work along relevant arm and leg channels. For example, if the patient has a Yang Ming frontal headache, work along the Stomach and Large Intestine meridians; if there is also Damp present then you may also be working on the Spleen and Lung Tai Yin channels. Stimulate your chosen distal points as you work along the channels.
- Do some work on the chest if the headaches are related to Damp, Phlegm, rebellious Qi, Wind invasions or Liver-Qi stagnation.
- Work on the abdomen for headaches related to digestive disharmony and for Qi, Blood and Kidney Xu.
- Work locally on the face and head to finish.

The treatment foundation routines for both the head and face and the neck and nape form an excellent framework for effective local work in the treatment of headaches. If the headaches are coming from an underlying Deficiency, the local work should be applied gently, taking your time over each part. If the headache is due to Excess, create stronger stimulation and apply the techniques briskly for a shorter period of time. In addition to this, add relevant points and techniques that may be applicable to the disharmony.

To help you plan a Tui na treatment for headaches, see Table 14.1 for some suggestions of useful techniques to consider including in the treatment of common patterns of disharmony.

Migraine exercise to show to patients

If done at the first signs of a migraine before the headache has come on, this can stop it developing fully. Sit in a quiet place on an upright chair. Take off your shoes and socks and put your feet flat on the floor. Keep your spine straight and place the backs of your hands on your thighs, fingers relaxed. Imagine a thermometer in each hand, and your palms becoming red hot. Try to make the gauge reach maximum. Think of heat moving down your arms from your head to your palms. Do this for about 5 minutes, then stimulate Liv3 and LI4 with Rou fa or pinching–grasping for several minutes on each side until the points ache strongly. Follow this by drinking a glass of water.

Headache case studies

Headache

Main complaint

Izzy, aged 15, was brought along for treatment by her Mum who I was treating for digestive and sinus problems at the time. She had been having a lot of headaches recently, at least once a week, and had fainted a couple of times at school. Her headaches were always on her forehead and were dull in nature; they were particularly bad the week after her period and when she was tired. They were better for rest. She had a poor appetite; I already knew from her Mum that Izzy did not eat well; she would not eat breakfast and often only had a sandwich or some chips for lunch at school; she had been vegetarian for the previous 2 years and ate very little fresh food. She was finding it difficult to concentrate at school and her Mum told me that she had become increasingly uncommunicative which was out of character. Izzy was very keen on sport and led a very busy life with lots of after-school activity.

Secondary complaints

Izzy's periods started when she was 12. Over the previous 18 months her periods had been very heavy; they lasted

Table 14.1 Suggestions for the treatment of headaches

Presenting disharmony	Useful treatment techniques
Wind-Cold	Gua sha or cupping along the Yang channels of the neck, nape and back Gua fa along the Governing Vessel and Bladder channel Tan bo fa and Na fa to the Bladder channel sinew in the neck, nape and back Kneading and nipping to Well points and Governing Vessel points Pinching–grasping the area of GB21 Clockwise palm Rou fa on Ren4 Ca fa on the back along the Bladder channel and across BL23 Yi zhi chan tui fa, anti-clockwise Rou fa and strong pinching–grasping for point stimulation
Wind-Heat	Gua sha or cupping along the Yang channels of the neck, nape and back Gua fa along the Governing Vessel and Bladder channel Nipping–grasping and kneading–nipping along the Governing Vessel and for stimulating points such as Du14, LI11 and GB20 Ca fa on the back along the Bladder channel Dredge the Yang channels with Na fa and Tui fa
Wind-Damp	Gua sha or cupping along the Yang channels of the neck, nape and back Pinching–grasping the Bladder channel sinew in the neck, nape and back Single-finger Ji dian fa on local head points, i.e. ST8, Du23 and Du20 Dredge the Yang channels with Na fa and Tui fa Pai fa and joined palm Ji fa to the back and limbs Zhen fa, Ji dian fa and Ca fa on the chest Palm Rou fa on Ren12

Table 14.1 Suggestions for the treatment of headaches—cont'd

Presenting disharmony	Useful treatment techniques
Liver-Yang rising	Gua sha along the Governing Vessel from Du16 to Du4, the Bladder channel from BL10 to BL23 and the Gallbladder channel from GB20 to GB21 Tui fa, Rou fa and kneading–pinching along the same channels Lifting–grasping along the spine from Du14 to the sacrum An fa on BL18 with intention on descending Qi and soothing Liver The basics of the chest and hypochondrium routine with an emphasis on Tui fa, Rou fa and pushing–pressing the supra- and infraclavicular fossas An fa on ST12 with the intention of descending Qi Tui fa to KD1 Ba shen fa to the neck Gua fa and Ma fa to the sides of the head Kneading–grasping and pulling the ears
Turbid Phlegm obstructing	Gun fa to the shoulders and back Ji dian fa and Yi zhi chan tui fa to the Back Shu points Forearm Rou fa to BL20 Forearm Rou fa over Ren12 and Ren6 coordinated with Gun fa, Pai fa and Ji dian fa down the Stomach channel Kneading–nipping PC6 with single-finger Ji fa on ST40 Apply the basic routine for the chest with an emphasis on An fa, Rou fa, Zhen fa and Ji dian fa; Rou fa or Zhen fa on Ren22 Pai fa and joined palm Ji fa on the back and limbs
Qi Deficiency	Tui fa, palm Rou fa and lifting–gasping along the Governing Vessel from the sacrum to the nape Clockwise Rou fa to stimulate Du4, Du14 and Du20 Pai fa to the vertex Ca fa to Du4 and Du14 Palm Rou fa, Mo fa and figure-of-eight Tui fa over the relevant Back Shu points Tui fa, Rou fa and Ca fa along the relevant Yin and Yang channels in the arms and legs Point stimulation with An fa, clockwise Rou fa and gentle Yi zhi chan tui fa Yin style holding and joining points such as ST36 and Ren12, LU9 and Ren17 Rou fa and tai chi Mo fa on the abdomen Warming palm, work with intention and holding over major points, Deficient organs and the affected areas on the head; work with breath and visualization Direct moxa to tonify points Indirect moxa to stimulate Du20 to raise the Yang
Blood Deficiency	Forearm Rou fa and palm Rou fa over BL14, BL17, BL20 and BL23 Figure-of-eight Tui fa around the relevant Back Shu points Gentle Tui fa, An fa and Rou fa on the chest Yin style holding and joining points Tui fa, Mo fa, Rou fa and Na fa along the Spleen, Liver, Lung and Pericardium channels focusing on the Ying Qi level Warming palm, work with intention and holding over major points, Deficient organs and the affected areas on the head; work with breath and visualization Tai chi Mo fa on the abdomen Palm Rou fa and Zhen fa over Ren4 Direct moxa to tonify points
Kidney Deficiency	Tui fa, Rou fa and Ya fa with the palm along the Bladder channel from the nape to the toe Moderate Gun fa for about 20 minutes along the Bladder channel concentrating on the lower back around the Kidney Back Shu points Forearm Rou fa, figure-of-eight Tui fa and Mo fa over BL23 and BL52 Ca fa over BL23 and BL52 Tui fa, Mo fa, Rou fa and Ca fa along the Kidney channels of the legs Forearm or palm Rou fa and Zhen fa to Ren4, Ren6 or Ren8 Warming palm over the kidneys, the back of the head and over the eyes

for 7 days and often they were painful at the beginning. She felt completely drained during and after her period, and had fainted towards the end of her last two periods.

Palpation and observation

Izzy was incredibly pale and looked very tired when I saw her initially.

Tongue

Her tongue was pale with orangey sides.

Pulse

Her pulse was Deep, Thready and Weak.

Diagnosis

The diagnosis was Qi and Blood Xu.

Treatment principle

This was to nourish Blood, invigorate Qi and raise Yang.

Treatment

With the patient seated

The head routine was applied with an emphasis on Tui fa, Mo fa and loose fist Pai fa at Du20.

With the patient lying prone

- Tui fa and palm Rou fa along the Governing Vessel from the sacrum to the nape and along the Bladder channel from the nape to the sacrum
- Lifting–grasping along the Governing Vessel from the sacrum to the nape 10 times
- Ca fa along the Governing Vessel and Bladder channel
- I then applied indirect moxa to Du14, BL17, BL19 and BL20 using a moxa stick with bird-pecking technique for about 2 minutes on each point
- Gentle Yin style An fa to the above Back Shu points, directing my attention and Qi down to the Ying Qi level

With the patient supine

- Tui fa and Rou fa along the Stomach, Spleen and Liver channels in the legs
- Indirect moxa on ST36 for 2 minutes
- An fa and Rou fa to stimulate ST36, SP6 and Liv8

On the abdomen

- Tui fa along the Stomach channel
- Palm Rou fa over Ren12, Ren6 and Ren4
- Tai chi Mo fa clockwise

On the face

- The foundation routine for the face working mainly around the forehead, eyes and ears
- Warming palm over her eyes and forehead
- Ji dian fa to Du20 to finish

Advice to the patient

After the first couple of treatments, Izzy came to see me on her own and I was able to talk to her in some depth about food and eating habits in terms of Chinese medicine. She immediately engaged with the concept of Qi and how Qi and Blood were produced from the food that we gave to our bodies. We talked about the extra demands that are put on our Qi and Blood when we engage in sport and how to build up these vital substances with food and regular eating patterns. I stressed the importance of breakfast and suggested that she always kept some fruit and nuts in her bag so that she could eat these throughout the day.

I also suggested that for the next couple of months she eased up with the extra sporting demands during her period.

Progress and subsequent treatments

I treated Izzy weekly for 8 weeks to see what progress we could make over two menstrual cycles. During this time she made a great effort with her diet and eating patterns; she started to eat breakfast, began to eat a lot more fresh fruit and vegetables and took a good packed lunch and plenty of fruit and nuts to school. With the weekly treatments and the changes that she made to her diet, things changed pretty quickly and by the end of the 8 weeks she was looking and feeling much better. There were no more headaches, no fainting and her energy and concentration were much improved. I continued to treat her fortnightly for the next 2 months, and 9 months later, I was giving her treatment occasionally only if she had a very demanding time coming up.

I have treated several cases similar to this and increasingly so over the past 4 years. I have found that teenagers respond very quickly to treatment with Tui na, much in the same way that babies and young children respond to pediatric Tui na.

Migraine

Main complaint

Fiona, aged 40, came for treatment to help with migraines. Her sister had been seeing me for acupuncture and had recommended that she come for treatment. Fiona was scared of needles and did not want acupuncture, but had heard from her sister that it might be possible to treat her migraines with massage instead.

Fiona had suffered with migraines since her early 20s; they had become increasingly worse over the previous 5 years. She had a migraine every month a day or two before her period and also if she was stressed or overworked. At the time she came to see me, she was having a migraine two or three times a month. They started with a feeling of stiffness in her neck and shoulders the day before. She had visual disturbance in the form of a green zig-zag light, usually in her left eye, and then the headache would come on, which she described as an intense throbbing sensation in her right temple. The headaches were accompanied by nausea and sometimes by vomiting and dizziness. The migraines lasted for 2 or 3 days.

Secondary complaints

Fiona's menstrual cycle was a regular 27 days. Her periods were very light and lasted for 3 days; she often felt dizzy after her period. She felt tired easily, had dry eyes and often experienced blurred vision. She said she always felt tight and achy in her neck and shoulders.

Palpation and observation

Fiona was generally very tight in her neck, shoulders and upper back. There was a tender knotted area directly over SJ15 on the left, and there was tenderness at GB20 and GB21 and the Huatuojiaji points from T1 to T7.

Tongue

Her tongue was red with lots of red points at the tip and there was no coating.

Pulse

Her pulse was generally Deep, Weak, Thin and slightly Quick, apart from the left middle position in her premenstrual week, which became Wiry.

Diagnosis

The diagnosis was Liver-Yang rising with underlying Liver-Yin Xu, and stagnation of Qi in the Tai Yang and Shao Yang channel sinews.

Treatment principle

This was to release and relax the Yang channel sinews in the neck and nape, soothe the Liver, descend rebellious Yang and nourish Liver-Yin.

As Fiona's migraines always came in the premenstrual phase of her cycle, I concentrated mainly on descending Yang, soothing the Liver and releasing the sinews in the second half of her cycle and focused on nourishing Yin in the postmenstrual week.

Treatment

With the patient seated

- I applied the area routine for the head

With the patient lying prone

- To help to release the Yang channel sinews, clear stagnation and descend Yang I started treatment with gua sha, working down the Governing Vessel from Du16 to Du4, the Bladder channel from BL10 to BL23 and the Gallbladder channel from GB20 to GB21. (In the first three treatments, a lot of red sha came to the surface; as she improved this gradually disappeared)
- Tui fa, Rou fa and pinching–grasping along the Governing Vessel, Bladder and Gallbladder channels in the neck, nape and back
- Kneading–nipping GB20 and Du14
- An fa and Rou fa to stimulate GB21 and SJ15
- Moving Yi zhi chan tui fa either side of the spine to stimulate the Huatuojiaji points from T1 to T7
- Double-handed Gun fa from the shoulders to the waist
- Forearm Rou fa to stimulate BL18 and BL23
- Kneading–grasping to release the muscles above and below the scapula
- Kneading–grasping and kneading–pinching down the Yang channels of the arms, releasing areas of congestion in her forearms as I found them
- Yi zhi chan tui fa to stimulate SJ5 and LI4
- Nian fa to the fingers
- Ca fa to KD1

With the patient supine

- Yi zhi chan tui fa to Liv3
- Mo fa along the Yin channels of the legs

On the chest

- Tui fa from Ren22 to Ren4 and across the chest
- An fa and Rou fa between the intercostal spaces
- Pushing–pressing the supraclavicular fossa
- Tui fa across the ribs

On the abdomen

- Tai chi Mo fa
- Palm Rou fa to Ren4
- Warming palm over Ren4

On the face

- Using the foundation routine for the face as the framework, concentrating on the areas of her forehead, temples, around her eyes and ears
- Warming palm over her eyes and temples

Advice to the patient

I showed Fiona how to apply gua sha to her neck and shoulders and suggested that she did this when she felt the pre-migraine stiffness in her neck coming on. I also showed her the migraine exercise described on page 166. I encouraged her to go back to yoga classes, which she had enjoyed in the past, to help her to relax and to give her some time out from her very busy work schedule.

Progress and subsequent treatments

Fiona responded well to Tui na. She came once a week for a month and then fortnightly for 5 months. By the end of the second month of treatment she was having one migraine a month premenstrually, her energy levels were picking up and she had not experienced any dizziness. She continued to improve and had no further premenstrual migraines from the fourth month of treatment. She found gua sha and the migraine exercise very useful as preventative measures and continues to use these if she feels any signs of a possible migraine. It is now several years since I started to treat Fiona; I still see her once every 2 or 3 months for preventative and maintenance treatment. She has a migraine on average once or twice a year if she has been overdoing things at work.

Hypertension

The patients that I tend to see in clinic with high blood pressure are stressed, middle-aged men and my elderly patients who are often very concerned about their blood pressure. I have found Tui na treatment of great benefit in the management of hypertension in both of these groups of patients.

As we know, hypertension can be caused by stress and is certainly worse for stress, so calming and soothing the Shen and the Qi is of great importance in treatment.

In elderly patients, the root of the problem is usually Deficiency of Kidney-Yin and sometimes both Kidney-Yin and Yang. Deficient Kidney-Yin cannot nourish Liver-Yin and consequently Liver-Yang becomes hyperactive and rebellious. The rebellious Yang can be accompanied by Phlegm and/or Wind.

In stressed, middle-aged patients, the root of the problem is usually a combination of lifestyle factors: too much alcohol and rich food, lack of exercise and rest combined with working too hard and stressful personal circumstances.

Depending on your diagnosis of the underlying disharmony, Tui na treatment usually involves:

- Calming and soothing the Shen, Qi and the Liver
- Descending rebellious Yang Qi
- Cooling and quelling Fire
- Nourishing Yin and supporting Yang
- Tonifying the Kidneys

- Supporting the Spleen and dredging and eliminating Damp and Phlegm

Special technique for lowering the blood pressure

This is a very useful simple technique that I was shown in the Tui na department at the Nanjing second affiliated hospital of traditional Chinese medicine.

Using a little talc as a massage medium, apply Tui fa with your thumbs from SJ17 to ST12 along the sterno-cleidomastoid muscles, for 5 minutes on each side. Effectively, you are mechanically lowering the blood pressure by pushing along the carotid artery and stimulating the carotid sinus, which sends a reflex response to the brain to lower the blood pressure.

General tips for treating hypertension

- To relax and soothe the patient, start treatment by doing some work on the patient's head and face using the basis of the foundation routine.
- Release the neck, nape and shoulders and stimulate any relevant points in these areas.
- Apply the special technique for lowering the blood pressure described above.
- Work on the back next; for example, apply gua sha to the Governing Vessel if the pulse is Full and Wiry and the patient has strong symptoms. Stimulate relevant points, channels and areas on the back.
- Work along relevant arm and leg channels and distal points with suitable techniques according to the disharmony.
- For elderly patients with Kidney Xu, apply gentle Yin style Tui na to the lower back, abdomen, channels and points to nourish the Yin. Remember that to nourish with Tui na, you need to work on an area for a relatively long period of time. For example, if you are applying gentle clockwise palm Rou fa to Ren4, you will be applying this for about 5 minutes. In Deficient cases, choose fewer points and areas to treat.
- Work on the chest if Phlegm is part of the problem.
- Work on the abdomen for all cases rooted in Deficiency.
- Finish with gentle work on the face.
- Stimulating GB30 with elbow Ya fa and KD1 with Rou fa is useful for all disharmonies.

To help you plan a Tui na treatment for hypertension, see Table 14.2 for some suggestions of useful techniques to consider including in the treatment of common patterns of disharmony.

Hypertension case study

To help to illustrate the treatment of hypertension with Tui na I have included the following case of a patient I treated in clinic.

Main complaint

David, aged 43, had been told by his GP that his blood pressure was too high. He had discussed with her that he would prefer not to take drugs and would like to try alternative methods first.

He had started working freelance 2 years previously and was constantly worried that work would dry up; this meant he over-compensated by saying yes to everything. This had spiralled out of control over the previous 6 months and he had found himself working 13-hour days on a regular basis. Things were difficult at home as he and his wife both worked from home and they had three young children. David told me that he had become slightly obsessed with taking his own blood pressure; he was taking it every morning and evening and noticed his systolic pressure was quite volatile. When his GP took his pressure, it was 160/85, and when he took his own pressure, the systolic ranged from 140 to 170.

He was very concerned that he was so easily stressed; the slightest thing could make him feel almost panic-stricken.

David's diet was not great: he was overweight and confessed to having a very sweet tooth, he drank coffee all day long and he ate a lot of dairy products. He used to play rugby but several knee injuries and his increased weight had a put a stop to that so he did not get any exercise. He spent hours in front of his computer and on the phone. David had a red face; he felt hot all the time and disliked hot weather. He said he knew when his pressure was up because he would get a throbbing temporal headache and feel extremely hot and agitated. His head often felt muzzy for a few days after this.

Secondary complaints

David complained of a very stiff neck. He was also bothered by Phlegm in the back of his throat.

Palpation and observation

David's neck and shoulder muscles were very tight.

Tongue

His tongue was swollen and red, especially at the sides and front, with a greasy yellow coating.

Pulse

His pulse was Quick and Wiry with a Slippery quality on the right.

Diagnosis

The diagnosis was Liver-Fire rebelling upwards with accumulated Phlegm.

Treatment principle

This was to quell the Fire, descend rebellious Yang, cool and soothe the Liver, calm the mind and eliminate Phlegm.

Treatment

With the patient seated

- Tui fa and Mo fa on his head
- Special technique for lowering the blood pressure

Table 14.2 Suggestions for the treatment of hypertension

Presenting disharmony	Useful treatment techniques
Liver-Fire blazing	Gua sha along the Governing Vessel from Du16 to Du4, the Bladder channel from BL10 to BL23 and the Gallbladder channel from GB20 to GB21
	Che fa or pinching–grasping along the Governing Vessel and Bladder channel in the back and along the Shao Yang and Yang Ming channels in the arms and legs and the Yin channels of the arms
	Tan bo fa along the Bladder channel sinew, stimulating the Back Shu points, focusing on the Liver Back Shu point
	Elbow Ya fa and Rou fa to GB30
	Kneading–nipping, nipping–grasping and strong Yi zhi chan tui fa to stimulate points
	Face routine to soothe and calm
	Rou fa to KD1
Accumulation of Phlegm	Head routine with an emphasis on Tui fa and Mo fa
	Gua sha with your nails over the ST8 area
	Tui fa and pinching–grasping the back along the Bladder channel
	Ya fa and Rou fa to stimulate GB30
	Pai fa and Ji fa on the back and limbs to disperse Phlegm
	Dredging the Yang Ming and Tai Yin channels along the arms and legs with Tui fa and kneading–grasping and Nian fa at the fingers and toes to dredge through to the extremities
	Chest and hypochondrium routine with an emphasis on Ji dian fa and Zhen fa
	Abdominal routine especially Tui fa, Rou fa, Mo fa and palm Pai fa
	Coordinated forearm Rou fa over Ren12 and Che fa to stimulate ST40 then Gun fa along the Stomach channel
Deficient Yin and hyperactive rebellious Yang	Head routine with emphasis on Tui fa and Mo fa
	Che fa to stimulate GB20 and GB21
	Lifting–grasping along the spine from Du14 to the sacrum
	An fa on BL18 with the intention of descending Qi and soothing Liver
	Ya fa and Rou fa to stimulate GB30
	Figure-of-eight Tui fa, Mo fa and palm Rou fa over the Kidney area
	Gentle Yin style point stimulation such as holding and joining points like BL23 and KD3
	Pushing–pressing BL40
	The basics of the chest and hypochondrium routine with an emphasis on Tui fa, Rou fa, Mo fa and pushing–pressing the supraclavicular fossa
	An fa on ST12 with the intention of descending Qi
	Tui fa or gentle Rou fa to stimulate KD1
	Face routine to finish
Kidney-Yin and Yang Xu	The basics of the head, neck and nape routines
	Tui fa, Rou fa and Na fa along the Bladder channel from the nape to the toe
	Coordinated technique Gun fa and forearm Rou fa, concentrating on the lower back around the Kidney Back Shu points
	Figure-of-eight Tui fa and Mo fa over BL23 and BL52
	Ca fa over BL23 and BL52
	Tui fa, Mo fa, Rou fa and Ca fa along the Kidney channels of the legs
	Tui fa or gentle Rou fa to stimulate KD1
	Forearm or palm Rou fa to Ren4 and Ren8
	Mo fa and Tui fa over the lower ribs
	Tai chi Mo fa on the abdomen
	Warming palm over the Kidneys, the back of the head and over the eyes

With the patient lying prone

- Gua sha along the Governing Vessel from Du16 to Du4, the Bladder channel from BL10 to BL23 and the Gallbladder channel from GB20 to GB21
- Nipping–grasping Du14 and pinching–grasping down the Governing Vessel to Du4 three times
- Kneading–nipping GB20 and kneading–pinching the neck along the Bladder and Gallbladder channels
- Tui fa down his back along the Bladder channel from the nape to the sacrum
- Pinching–grasping along the Bladder channel from the nape to the sacrum
- Double-handed Gun fa to release his shoulders and upper back

- Tan bo fa along the Bladder channel from the nape to the waist
- Strong Yi zhi chan tui fa on BL18 and BL20
- Strong Ya fa and Rou fa on GB30 until the point was very hot
- Pai fa and Tui fa down his back, arms and legs to dissipate and dredge Phlegm
- Thumb Rou fa to stimulate KD1

With the patient supine

- Tui fa and pinching–grasping along the Stomach and Spleen channels in his legs
- Yi zhi chan tui fa to stimulate ST36, and single-finger Ji dian fa to stimulate ST40

- Yi zhi chan tui fa to stimulate Liv2 and thumb Rou fa to stimulate SP6
- Pai fa along the Yin and Yang channels of the legs
- Tui fa and pinching–grasping along the Yin and Yang channels of the arms
- The basics of the face routine plus Gua fa to stimulate ST8
- Kneading and grasping the sternocleidomastoid
- Pushing–pressing the supraclavicular fossa
- Tui fa, Rou fa and Ji dian fa on the chest
- Tui fa and Mo fa on the ribs and abdomen

To finish

- Holding KD1

Advice to the patient

We discussed diet and exercise at some length. I knew it was essential not to stress him out further by giving him too much to do or by suggesting things that it was highly unlikely that he would initially be able to achieve. So, I kept it simple and suggested he take a half hour walk each day to begin to build up his fitness levels and get away from his computer and phone. I suggested he drank more water by replacing half his cups of coffee with glasses of water and asked him to cut down his dairy and sugar intake and to increase his intake of fish, fruit and vegetables. I also suggested that he stopped taking his own

blood pressure for the time being and that he wait for a period of 3 months when he was due to see his GP again for a check-up.

Progress and subsequent treatments

David was very committed to his weekly Tui na treatments; he came once a week for 3 months and over this time he made some very important changes to his daily routine. He really took to his walks, which he increased to an hour a day after lunch. He found they relaxed him and helped him to think more clearly. He made several changes to his diet including reducing coffee to one cup in the morning, cutting out cheese and strictly limiting his sugar intake. He also made the decision to rent an office rather than continuing to work from home; this made it easier for him to regulate his working hours and significantly took the pressure off at home.

After 6 weeks I noticed a marked change in his pulses; they were slower and less Full and Wiry. By this stage he was feeling a whole lot better in himself, he was able to deal with things more calmly and he generally felt more relaxed. At the end of the 3-month period, when he went back to see his GP, his blood pressure was 137/82 and he was having no more hypertensive symptoms.

David now sees me once every few months in general and more frequently if he feels he needs to.

CHAPTER **15**

Coughs, colds and asthma

Common colds and coughs

Tui na is a particularly effective form of treatment for acute Exterior invasions because of its ability to clear, release and disperse at the Wei Qi level. It produces excellent results in the treatment of coughs and colds, both at the acute stage and when the symptoms are lingering and leaving the patient tired, stiff, achy and generally run down.

Depending on your diagnosis and the level at which the presenting disharmony is expressing itself, treatment of coughs and colds usually involves a combination of the following:

- Expelling external pathogenic factors, releasing the Exterior and dispersing obstructed Wei Qi
- Descending rebellious Lung-Qi
- Eliminating Damp and Phlegm and dredging the channels
- Tonifying Lung-Qi
- Nourishing Lung-Yin
- Tonifying the Kidneys
- Tonifying the Spleen

General tips for treating coughs and colds

- If you are treating an acute Exterior invasion affecting the Wei Qi level, apply cupping or gua sha before Tui na treatment.
- Work on the patient's head, neck, nape and upper back first, using the area foundation routines as your framework.
- Work along the Governing Vessel to clear Heat or to scatter Cold.
- For Exterior invasions, work along the Bladder and Small Intestine Tai Yang channels towards the Jing Well points. Focus on stirring up the pathogens at the Wei Qi level and then dredging them out of the body through the Jing Well points by working along the channels and stimulating points with techniques like Tui fa, Rou fa and compound versions of Rou fa.
- If the patient has a cough, remember to work on their back before you work on their chest. Use the area foundation routine for the chest as a framework for treatment in this area.
- If the patient has a lot of Phlegm use striking techniques on the back and limbs and Ji dian fa on chest points.
- If the patient has a chronic cough with Damp Phlegm, work on the abdomen and Spleen and Stomach channels of the legs to support and tonify the Spleen-Qi.
- To treat Deficiency such as Lung- and Kidney-Yin Xu and Lung- and Spleen-Qi Xu, use gentle yin style work on points, channels and key areas such as around relevant Back Shu points and on the chest and abdomen.
- Finish treatment by working on the face using the basis of the area routine. If the patient has a headache and their sinuses are very blocked, spend at least 15 minutes working on their face and they will feel a lot better.

To help you to plan a Tui na treatment for coughs and colds, see Table 15.1 for some suggestions of techniques to consider including in the treatment of the most common patterns of disharmony.

Table 15.1 Suggestions for the treatment of common colds and coughs

Presenting disharmony	Useful treatment techniques
Wind-Cold	Cupping over BL12 and generally to the upper back, or gua sha along the Yang channels of the neck, nape and back
	Gua fa along the Governing Vessel and Bladder and Small Intestine channels
	Ca fa along the Governing Vessel and either side of the spine until hot
	Tui fa and Mo fa on the head
	Pinching–grasping and plucking–grasping the neck, nape and back
	Pinching–grasping the area of GB21
	Kneading and nipping the Bladder and Small Intestine Jing Well points
	Rou fa and kneading–grasping to dredge along the Bladder and Small Intestine channels
	Gun fa to the upper back, nape and shoulders
	Anti-clockwise thumb Rou fa or strong Yi zhi chan tui fa to stimulate relevant points such as GB20 and BL12
	Foundation routine for the face
	Apply the techniques strongly
Wind-Heat	Cupping over BL12 and Du14 and generally to the upper back, or gua sha along the Yang channels of the neck, nape and back
	Gua fa, Tui fa and Ca fa along the Governing Vessel and Bladder channel from the nape to the sacrum
	Nipping–grasping and kneading–nipping along the Governing Vessel
	Tui fa and Mo fa on the head
	Pinching–grasping and kneading–grasping the neck, nape and shoulders
	Kneading–nipping points such as LI4 and SJ5
	Dredge the channels with compound versions of Rou fa and Tui fa
	Use the foundation area routine for the chest with an emphasis on Tui fa, Rou fa and Ji dian fa
	Use the foundation area routine for the face
	Apply the techniques moderately
Wind-Cold-Damp	As for Wind-Cold plus:
	Zhen fa, Ji dian fa and Ba shen fa on the neck
	Pai fa and joined palm Ji fa to the back and limbs
	Zhen fa, Ji dian fa and Ca fa on the chest
	Thumb Rou fa and forearm Rou fa to stimulate BL20 and BL21
	Palm or forearm Rou fa on Ren12
	Nipping–kneading the Stomach channel from ST36 to ST41
Wind-Damp Heat	As for Wind-Heat plus:
	Kneading–grasping and lifting–grasping the ears
	Ji dian fa and Zhen fa on the chest
	Pinching–grasping, kneading–pinching and nipping–kneading the Large Intestine channels from LI11 to LI4, the San Jiao channel from SJ10 to SJ4, the Stomach channel from ST36 to ST41 and the Gallbladder channel from GB34 to GB40
Phlegm-Heat in the Lungs	Cupping over BL13, Du14 and SI11 and generally on the upper back and shoulders
	Stimulate BL13, BL17 and BL20 with Rou fa, Yi zhi chan tui fa and Ji dian fa
	Release the paraspinal muscles from C7 to T12 with Rou fa, Gun fa, and moving Yi zhi chan tui fa and Tan bo fa
	Zhen fa and middle-finger Rou fa to stimulate Ren22
	Foundation area routine for the chest and hypochondrium with an emphasis on Zhen fa, Ji dian fa, pushing–pressing the supra- and infraclavicular fossas
	Palm Rou fa and Zhen fa along the lateral side of the ribcage
	Dredge the Lung, Large Intestine, Stomach and Spleen channels with compound versions of Na fa and Tui fa
	Ji fa, Ji dian fa and Pai fa to the back, arms and legs to dissipate the Phlegm
	Whisking–sweeping the upper back and ribs
Damp Phlegm in the Lungs	Cupping along the Bladder channel from BL13 to BL20
	Tui fa and Ca fa on the back from the nape to the sacrum along and horizontally across the Bladder channel until hot
	Rou fa, Gun fa, pinching–grasping and Ji dian fa along the Bladder channel in the back and down the legs
	Ji dian fa, Yi zhi chan tui fa and Zhen fa for point stimulation
	Palm or forearm Rou fa over the Stomach and Spleen Back Shu points
	Pai fa and joined palm Ji fa on the back
	Zhen fa and middle-finger Rou fa to stimulate Ren22
	Chest and hypochondrium routine with an emphasis on Tui fa from Ren22 to Ren17, Ji dian fa, Zhen fa and pushing and pressing the supra- and infraclavicular fossas
	Ca fa across the chest and along the Lung and Spleen channels
	Zhen fa and palm Pai fa to the lateral sides of the ribcage
	Palm Rou fa to Ren12 plus thumb Rou fa to ST36
	Tui fa and Mo fa to the abdomen
	Tui fa, kneading–grasping, Gun fa, Ji dian fa and Pai fa to the Yin and Yang channels of the arms and legs

Presenting disharmony	Useful treatment techniques
Lung-Qi Deficiency	Tui fa and Rou fa along the Bladder channel
	Ca fa along the Bladder channel and across BL13
	Gentle An fa and Rou fa to BL13 and BL43
	Figure-of-eight Tui fa around BL13 and BL43
	Warming and holding with the palms over BL13 and BL43
	Apply direct moxa to chosen points such as BL13, LU9 and Ren12
	Tui fa, Mo fa, gentle Rou fa and Ca fa to the Lung and Spleen channels
	Palm Rou fa and Mo fa to Ren12
	Chest and hypochondrium routine with an emphasis on gentle An fa, Rou fa and Tui fa
	Tui fa, Rou fa and Mo fa to the abdomen
	Warming and holding with your palms on the chest over points such as Ren17 and LU1
Lung-Yin Xu	Tui fa and Rou fa along the Bladder channel
	Gentle An fa and Rou fa to BL13 and BL43
	Figure-of-eight Tui fa around BL13 and BL43
	Warming and holding with the palms over BL13 and BL43
	Holding and connecting LU7 and KD6 to open the Ren Mai channel with your attention at the level of the Yuan Qi. When the points feel open and warm, apply Zhen fa
	Tui fa, Mo fa and Rou fa along the Yin channels of the arm and legs
	Stimulate points on the Lung, Spleen and Kidney channels with gentle An fa, Rou fa, Yi zhi chan tui fa, Zhen fa or holding and connecting two points
	Tui fa along the Ren Mai channel from Ren2 to Ren12
	Palm Rou fa and tai chi Mo fa over Ren4
	Foundation area routine for the chest with an emphasis on gentle Tui fa, An fa and Rou fa
	Holding with your palms on the chest over major points such as LU1
Lung- and Kidney-Yin Xu	As for Lung-Yin Xu plus:
	Moderate Gun fa on the lower back around the Kidney Back Shu points
	Forearm Rou fa, figure-of-eight Tui fa and Mo fa over BL23 and BL52
	Ca fa over BL23 and BL52
	Holding with your palms over the kidneys and over Ren4

Coughs and colds case studies

To help illustrate the treatment of common colds and coughs two cases of patients I have treated follow.

Cough

Main complaint

Brenda, aged 48, came in to see me with what she described as a dry irritating cough. I had treated her on several occasions before for hot flushes, night sweats and lower backache. She was an actress and often away from home so I had not seen her for 5 months.

About a month before she had had a bad cold with a productive cough and yellow phlegm. Since the cold symptoms had gone she had been left with this dry cough, which was worse in the afternoon and evening. Her throat felt dry all the time, her voice was husky and weak and she was constantly sipping water. She was very worried about her voice, as she had some filming work a fortnight from then.

Secondary complaints

Since having the cold, her energy levels had been low and she felt very tired, particularly in the late afternoon and early evening. Her hot flushes and night sweats had returned with a vengeance, her lower back ached and her shoulders and upper back felt uncomfortable and tight.

Palpation and observation

On palpation I noticed that Brenda was much tighter than usual in her trapezius, rhomboids and generally through her paraspinal muscles. There was marked tenderness at BL43, BL52 and the Huatuojiaji points from T2 to T7. She looked and felt Empty and Weak in her lower back around L5 where she felt vulnerable.

Tongue

Her tongue was dry and red towards the front with several small irregular cracks in the Lung area and no coating.

Pulse

Her pulse was Empty, Weak and slightly Quick.

Diagnosis

The diagnosis was Lung- and Kidney-Yin Xu.

Treatment principle

This was to nourish Lung- and Kidney-Yin, clear Empty Heat, descend the Lung-Qi and stop the cough.

Treatment

With the patient prone

I started treatment with empty cupping. I applied eight medium-sized cups along the Bladder channel from BL12 to BL23, keeping them moving on and off her body constantly for about 4 minutes to help to relax her muscles and invigorate her Qi without draining her.

Tui na treatment consisted of:

- Palm Tui fa along the Bladder channel from BL12 to BL60 and then across her back from the nape to the sacrum
- Kneading–grasping GB21 on the side nearest to me, coordinated with Rou fa down the Bladder channel on the opposite side; three times on each side
- Gentle to moderate double-handed Gun fa across her nape and shoulders and along the Bladder channel to the level of BL23, releasing the trapezius, rhomboids and paraspinals
- Moderate Gun fa on her lower back around BL23 and BL52 coordinated with Tui fa and gentle slow An fa down her legs along the Bladder channel
- Mo fa and figure-of-eight Tui fa around BL23 and BL52 coordinated with Gun fa down the backs of her legs along the Bladder channel; Brenda was very open and easy to work with and I asked her to breathe into her kidney area and to visualize them filling with deep blue energy
- Mo fa and figure-of-eight Tui fa around BL13 and BL43; I asked her to visualize a white light filling her lungs
- An fa and clockwise Rou fa very gently to stimulate BL13, BL43, BL23 and BL52
- To finish the work on her back I held the areas of BL13 and then BL23 with my palms for about 3 minutes in each place, visualizing Moon Qi nourishing her Lung- and Kidney-Yin

With the patient supine

- Holding and connecting LU7 on the right and KD6 on the left to open the Ren Mai with my attention at the level of her Yuan Qi; when the points felt open I applied gentle Zhen fa with my middle finger to the points, focusing gently on sending the vibration through to the Yuan level and nourishing her Yin
- Tui fa, Mo fa and Rou fa along the Yin channels of her arm and legs focusing on the Lung and Kidney channels
- Gentle clockwise Rou fa on KD3 and LU9

On her chest

- Tui fa from Ren22 to Ren17 and from the sternum across LU1 and LU2
- An fa and Rou fa gently along the intercostal spaces
- Kneading–grasping the pectoral muscles gently and softly
- Gentle clockwise Rou fa to stimulate LU1 while holding LU9 and intending and directing a connection between them
- Palm Rou fa over Ren4

Advice to the patient

I showed her how to apply some simple self-massage to her lower back, abdomen and chest and how to stimulate LU9 and KD3 with Rou fa. I suggested she did this every day. I also suggested that she drank plenty of fresh pear juice and, if possible, to lie down in the late afternoon for half an hour and rest.

Progress and subsequent treatments

I treated Brenda every other day for three treatments and by the time I saw her for her fourth treatment 4 days later, the cough had gone, and much to her relief her voice was back to normal. Her energy was also much better, as was the general muscular stiffness and lower backache. The hot flushes and night sweats had also started to improve again. I continued with two further treatments before she went away, varying the points to address the hot flushes and night sweating.

Common cold

Main complaint

Suzy, aged 35, is a regular patient of mine, who generally comes for maintenance treatments of a lower back problem I had treated in the past. Whenever she has a cold she comes to see me as soon as possible. On this occasion she had been having strong acute symptoms for 24 hours and she was feeling very rough. She was sneezing, had a very sore throat and a tickly cough, chills and fever, upper body aches, an aversion to cold weather and a headache. When she blew her nose there was yellow mucus and she was more thirsty than usual.

Palpation and observation

Her back, neck and head felt very hot to the touch.

Tongue

Her tongue was always slightly red but was more so on this occasion, especially at the front. Her tongue coating was thicker than usual and was slightly yellow.

Pulse

Her pulse was Floating and Rapid.

Diagnosis

Acute Exterior invasion of Wind-Heat.

Treatment principle

This was to release the Exterior, expel Wind, clear Heat, and help Wei Qi to disperse and Lung-Qi to descend.

Treatment

With the patient prone

- I started treatment with cupping. I applied seven cups in total, over Du14, BL12, BL14 and SI11. I left these in place for 15 minutes
- After I removed the cups I applied a little white flower balm to her back and began to work along the Governing Vessel and Bladder channel from her nape to her sacrum with Tui fa, Gua fa and Ca fa
- I applied anti-clockwise Rou fa with my thumbs to stimulate BL12 and nipping–kneading to stimulate Du14

- I continued with nipping–kneading along the Governing Vessel three times
- I worked on her neck and nape along the Bladder and Gallbladder channels with Tui fa, Rou fa, pinching–grasping and plucking–grasping. I stimulated BL10 and GB20 with kneading–nipping and GB21 with pinching–grasping
- I then opened and dredged the Bladder and Small Intestine channels with Tui fa, kneading–grasping and kneading–pinching, and as I reached her feet and hands, I moved to kneading–nipping. I opened the Jing Well points, BL67 and SI1 with kneading–nipping and focused on dredging the pathogens out of the channels and through those points
- I applied Nian fa to all her fingers and toes

With the patient supine

- I worked along the Lung, Large Intestine and San Jiao channels with Tui fa, kneading–grasping and kneading–nipping, stimulating points as I worked through the channels. I stimulated LI11 and LI5 simultaneously with kneading–grasping, SJ5 and LI4 with Yi zhi chan tui fa and LU11 with kneading–nipping
- On her chest I applied Tui fa from Ren22 to Ren17, and across her chest horizontally Rou fa to the intercostal spaces and dredged through the arm channels again

On the face

I used the foundation area routine for the face to finish.

Advice to the patient

I advised Suzy to take Echinacea, extra vitamin C and to drink plenty of water and honey and lemon. I told her to rest as much as possible and not to go into work until she felt better. I asked her to come and see me in 2 days.

Progress and subsequent treatments

When I saw Suzy 2 days later she was much better; she had taken my advice and went to bed straight after the treatment I gave her. She told me that she woke that night covered in sweat, went back to sleep and when she woke the next day she felt a lot better in herself. She no longer had chills and fever or body aches, but her throat was still slightly sore and she had a tickly, dry cough. Her pulses were still too Quick and she still felt too hot on her back. I treated her again in a similar manner to that described above but used gua sha along the Governing Vessel and Bladder channel instead of cupping.

I saw Suzy a week later and she was back to her normal self.

Asthma

I have found Tui na to be very useful and effective as a form of treatment for asthma, both during a period of acute attacks and between the attacks. As well as addressing the underlying energetic disharmonies associated with asthma, Tui na excels at releasing the muscular and emotional holding patterns and structural rigidity associated with asthmatic patients and helps to correct and improve their breathing.

During attacks

Treatment focuses on:

- Calming the asthma
- Releasing the obstructed Wei Qi
- Expelling the invading pathogenic factors
- Resolving and dredging Phlegm
- Descending the Lung-Qi
- Relaxing the muscles of the neck, shoulders, chest and upper back
- Facilitating the movement of the diaphragm and ribcage
- Calming the mind

Between attacks

Treatment focuses on:

- Tonifying the Lungs, Spleen and Kidneys
- Strengthening Wei Qi
- Resolving Phlegm
- Releasing the muscles, particularly the trapezius, rhomboids, paraspinals, pectorals, intercostals, diaphragm, hips and jaw
- Encouraging correct intercostal diaphragmatic breathing

During acute attacks

- Work with the patient seated.
- Stimulate extra point Dingchaun on both sides with strong thumb Rou fa or Yi zhi chan tui fa for 5 minutes.
- Stimulate BL13 with strong thumb Rou fa or Yi zhi chan tui fa for 3 minutes. Release the neck, nape and shoulders with techniques like Gun fa, kneading–grasping and pinching–grasping.
- Stimulate LU6 with strong An fa and Rou fa or Yi zhi chan tui fa for 3–5 minutes on each side.
- Apply the seated work described below.
- Do a little gentle work on the face using the basics of the face routine to help to calm the Shen.
- Finish with warming palm over GB21 thinking of Lung-Qi descending.

Between acute attacks

- Release muscular tension and structural rigidity and help to improve the patient's breathing by using the methods described below.
- Tonify the Lungs, Spleen and Kidneys by applying techniques like figure-of-eight Tui fa and Mo fa over the Back Shu points, tai chi Mo fa on the abdomen,

Tui fa, Mo fa, gentle Rou fa and Ca fa to the channels and gentle Rou fa or holding and connecting chosen points.

General tips for treating asthma

Use cupping on the upper back and shoulders before applying Tui na. Cupping can be applied both during periods when the acute attacks are frequent and in between the attacks.

Releasing muscular tension and structural rigidity and facilitating breathing

This is an essential part of the long-term treatment of asthma. I have found the following approach invaluable for releasing the muscular tension and rigidity associated with asthma and for helping to improve the patient's breathing.

With the patient seated

- Release the neck and nape using the area foundation routine as the basis for this
- Release the trapezius and rhomboid muscles with Rou fa and Gun fa
- Knead and grasp above and below the scapula
- Push and press the supraclavicular fossa
- Apply thumb Rou fa to the Huatuojiaji points from T1 to T7, from BL11 to BL17 and BL41 to BL46. Follow with moving Yi zhi chan tui fa, Tan bo fa and five-finger Ji dian fa along the same lines
- Apply Rou fa with the heels of your palms to the SI11 and LU1/2 area to release the pectoral muscles at the front and the scapular muscles at the back
- Dredge the stagnation down the arm channels with compound versions of Na fa and Rou fa

With the patient prone

- Apply Ca fa with the ulnar edge of your palms either side of the spine
- Double-handed Gun fa between the shoulder blades, focusing around BL13 and BL43
- Elbow Tui fa and Tan bo fa along the paraspinal muscles
- Simultaneously work on one shoulder and the opposite hip releasing the muscles with Rou fa, kneading–grasping and pinching–grasping; stimulate SI11 and GB30; dredge the stagnation along the arm and leg channels

With the patient on their side

The ribcage in asthmatic patients is rigid and hardly moves. A key part of treatment is to release the ribcage and facilitate correct breathing, as follows:

- Tui fa and palm Rou fa along the lateral side of the ribs
- With one hand at the front of the ribcage and one behind, move and release the ribs and intercostal muscles by pushing the ribcage back and forth between your hands, working up and down the ribcage
- Stretch the ribcage by holding under the patient's shoulder with one hand and their iliac crest with the other hand and pulling your hands away from each other
- Apply An fa with the heel of your palm from the axilla to the bottom of the ribcage; encourage the patient to breathe into their ribcage, apply your pressure as they exhale and release as they inhale; encourage them to try and push your hand away on the inhalation
- Use palm Zhen fa along the ribs, encouraging the patient to breathe into the vibration
- Apply forearm Rou fa to GB30 and elbow Ya fa to SI11

With the patient supine

- Apply the area foundation routine for the chest and hypochondrium, concentrating on releasing the pectoral muscles and the intercostal spaces
- Standing to one side of your patient, put your hands on either side of the ribcage and continue to release the ribs and intercostals by pushing and pulling the ribcage between your hands, working up and down the ribcage
- Using the ulnar edge of your palms under your patient's ribcage, use Rou fa to release the diaphragm, thinking of drawing it down towards the navel
- To help to release the diaphragm and improve the function of the lungs, work under the ribs, moving gradually from the area of Liv13 on the right to Liv13 on the left using An fa and Rou fa with both thumbs; work with your patient's breath, applying pressure as they exhale and releasing as they inhale
- The masseter muscles are often locked and tight in patients with asthma. Release the jaw by stimulating local points such as ST5 and ST6 with Rou fa and work along the jaw line with kneading–grasping
- Finish by applying palm Rou fa to Ren12 and Ren4

In terms of other suggestions for the treatment of the main patterns of disharmony associated with asthma you may find it useful to refer back to Table 15.1 for suggested techniques in the treatment of common colds and coughs, as the patterns associated with asthma are very similar.

CHAPTER **16**

Combining acupuncture and Tui na in practice

The majority of people who are currently studying Tui na are either already acupuncturists or are studying acupuncture and Tui na at the same time. These students frequently ask me how to approach the combination of these two therapies in practice. I work with this combination a great deal and find it practical, satisfying and clinically highly effective.

While writing this book I had the pleasure to meet the very experienced Dr Yang from Beijing who has over 60 years of experience working with this combination. Now in his late 80s and still a keen and dedicated practitioner of both disciplines, Dr Yang told me that in his experience, the combination of the two therapies was more effective than using either one in isolation, and treating patients with both acupuncture and Tui na produces better and faster results. I am inclined to agree. His method is always to give his patients acupuncture first and retain the needles for 15–20 minutes and then to remove the needles and apply 15–20 minutes of Tui na.

Dr Yang's method represents one very straightforward and effective way of working. I have met other practitioners who prefer to apply Tui na first and to give acupuncture treatment after this. I use both of these methods depending on the circumstances. For example, if a patient is very nervous of needles then I am more likely to give them some Tui na first. After 15 minutes of Tui na they will be more relaxed and able to accept and receive acupuncture treatment. So simply applying one therapy after another is one option. A few more suggestions for how to combine the two follow.

Applying Tui na while the needles are retained

This is the method that I use most frequently. There are several options:
- Needle the local area and apply Tui na distally. For example, if you are treating a patient with lower backache, first of all needle the points that you want to stimulate in the local lower back area and retain them. While the needles are in place you can work with Tui na along the Bladder channel sinew in the leg, stimulating distal points, dredging the channel and releasing areas of congestion and stagnation.
- Needle distally and apply Tui na locally. For example, this is very useful when patients have digestive and gynecological problems. Needle the chosen points according to your patient's disharmony, minus any abdominal points. While the needles are retained, work with Tui na on your patient's abdomen. This is a very powerful way of working if the patient's problem is manifesting in the Lower or Middle Jiao. I have found this method particularly effective for poor digestion, irritable bowel syndrome, menstrual problems and fertility issues.
- For patients who are nervous, stressed or suffering with insomnia, headaches, sinus problems or common colds, needle your chosen points leaving out any head or face points and simply try applying the Tui na area foundation routine for the face while the needles are retained. Patients generally love this.

Applying non-retained acupuncture during Tui na treatment

I have found this useful in the treatment of muscular skeletal conditions. As you work along the channels with Tui na, if you find areas that are particularly congested and stagnant, needle the area and apply Zhen fa with the needle for 30–60 seconds, focusing your attention on sending the vibration deeply into the point and along the channel. Then remove the needle and continue to disperse and dredge the channel with Tui na. This method helps to disperse very stubborn chronic stagnation of Qi and Blood.

These are just some suggestions. Try them and see what works for you.

Resources and further reading

Resources

UK Register of Tui na Chinese Massage (UKRTCM)
Website: **www.ukrtcm.org**

Tui na training

Recommended courses in the UK are presently offered at:

City College of Acupuncture
55 East Road
London
N1 6AH
Tel: 0207 253 1133
Website: **www.citycollegeofacupuncture.com**

University of Westminster
115 New Cavendish Street
London W1M 8JS
Tel: 0207 911 5000
Website: **www.westminster.ac.uk**

Contact the UK Register of Tui na Chinese Massage for up-to-date information on courses being offered in the UK.

Qigong

Shaolin Temple UK
207a Junction Road
Tufnell Park
London N19 5QA
Tel: 0207 7687 8333
Website: **www.shaolintempleuk.org**

Chris Chappeli
Website: **www.realtaoism.com**

Master Wu
Website: **www.masterwu.net**

Suppliers of moxa, cups, gua sha tools and basic external herbal massage media

Shulan UK Ltd
514 Parrs Wood Road
Didsbury
Manchester M20 5QA
Tel: 0161 488 1233
Website: **www.shulan.uk.com**

Mayway (UK) Ltd
19 Progress Way
Croydon
London CR0 4XD
Tel: 0208 688 8286
Website: **www.maywayuk.co.uk/store/stage/general**

Harmony Medical Distribution Ltd
629 High Road
Leytonstone
London E11 4PA
Tel: 0800 092 8123
Website: **www.harmonymedical.co.uk**

Oxford Medical Supplies Ltd
Unit 21
Langstone Priory Mews
Station Road
Kingham
Oxton
OX7 6UP
Tel: 0800 975 8111
Website: **www.oxfordmedical.co.uk**

DongBang AcuPrime Ltd
1 Forrest Units
Hennock Road East
Marsh Barton
Exeter
EX2 8RU
Tel: 0139 282 9500
Website: **www.acuprime.com**

Further information

For further information about Classical Chinese Medicine:

Association for Traditional Studies
Telephone: 828 398 0667
Email: **ats@traditionalstudies.org**
Website: **www.traditionalstudies.org**

For further information about the work of Janice Walton-Hadlock and the use of Yin style Tui na in the treatment of Parkinson's disease, contact:

The Parkinson's Recovery Project
343 Soquel Avenue
413 Santa Cruz
CA 95062, USA
Email: **pdinfo@cruzio.com**
Website: **www.pdrecovery.org**

For further information about Tui na including postgraduate training you may contact the author at:
Email: **sarah@healingpath.co.uk**
Website: **www.healingpath.co.uk**

Further information on herbs can be obtained from:
Website: **www.taohealingarts.com**

Further reading

Chinese massage

Guocai, W., Yali, F. and Zhang, G. (1990) *Chinese Massage* (Ed. Engin, Z.) Shanghai: Publishing House of Shanghai College of Traditional Chinese Medicine.

Hongzhu, J. (2005) *Chinese Tuina (Massage).* Shanghai: Publishing House of Shanghai University of Traditional Chinese Medicine

Hui, J. L. and Xiang, J. Z. (1987) *Pointing Therapy: a Chinese Traditional Therapeutic Skill.* Shangdon: Shangdon Science and Technology Press.

Pritchard, S. (2015) *Chinese Massage Manual* (2nd ed.). London: Singing Dragon.

Chinese Massage Therapy (1990) (Ed. Chengman, S.) Shangdong: Shangdong Science and Technology Press.

Ya-Li, F. (1994) *Chinese Pediatric Massage Therapy.* Boulder, CO: Blue Poppy Press

Qigong

Cohen, K. S. (1997) *The Way of Qigong.* New York: Ballantine Books.

Johnson, J. A. (2010) *Chinese Medical Qigong Therapy.* California: The International Institute of Medical Qigong.

Chinese Qigong (1990) Shanghai: Publishing House of Shanghai College of Traditional Chinese Medicine

Kit, W. K. (1996) *The Art of Chi Kung.* Shaftesbury: Element Books Inc

Cupping, Gua sha and Moxibustion

Chirali, I. Z. (2007) *Cupping Therapy* (2nd ed.). Edinburgh: Churchill Livingstone.

Nielsen, A. (1995) *Gua Sha: A Traditional Technique for Modern Practice.* Edinburgh: Churchill Livingstone.

Wilcox, L. (2009) *Moxibustion: A Modern Clinical Handbook.* Monrovia CA: Blue Poppy Press

Wilcox, L. (2008) *Moxibustion: The Power of Mugwort Fire.* Monrovia CA: Blue Poppy Press

Index

Please note that f represents figure and t represents table.